I.S HEALING SYSTEM™

A guide to understanding yourself

5 simple steps to releasing pain, stress and suffering

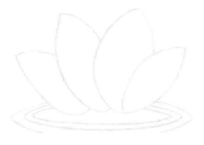

Adriana Kahrs

I dedicate this book to you my beloved reader, hoping that my life experiences and teaching will help you to have a more beautiful, loving and healthy life.

ACKNOWLEDGEMENTS

I would like to express my gratitude to My Own Inner Self, who allowed the information for this book to become a reality, to my life that I love and I am so grateful for each minute I have. My gratitude also goes to my dearest friends, Rod, Charlotte, Sara and Dev who helped me to structure this book.

Also, I want to say thank you to each one of my beloved clients who have provide so much insight, affection and wisdom.

FOREWORD

I got to know Adriana at a public speaking event where she was telling a story about a woman that had a couple of challenges in life. She addressed a specific night in the life of a young lady.

"Tick Tock, Tick Tock ….I heard footsteps, Tick, Tock, Tick Tock ".

She was telling this story in a way that was more than captivating, it felt very genuine and authentic. Referring to it as being intriguing would be an understatement. Later, I learned it was not just a story but it was her story.

This book is telling her story and believe me, she has quite a story to tell. So, is this then merely an autobiography of a Colombian girl that crossed the pond and started a life in Europe? No, every single fragment she describes tangles into "a discovery" towards her goal in life. While repressing her "gifts" at first, because they were perceived as not appropriate, she internally grew better in understanding the dynamics of people and more specifically in getting to the bottom of what makes people worrying or sick.

While she describes the lessons learned or skills developed in every stage of her life, as a reader you are challenged to self-reflect and compelled to turn the pages and read on, eager to find out more. The book is full of little gems that add up to Adriana's version of the holy grail or at least the closest she could get to it, for now.

Her 5 step system helps you to recognise difficulties that you are having which are preventing you finding inner peace and from identifying your quest in life, blocking your personal development and happiness.

After being able to label these subjects in the first step you will be flowing through the different steps in an upward motion which should result in an absolute feeling of "being you" in the most satisfying way. As always, it is about taking action, follow the steps, execute them and you will feel the transformation within, and around you.

I am so glad we've crossed roads as Adriana is a very inspirational strong woman capable of adding true value to one's life. I can't wait to learn new things from her and follow her future discoveries and the further development of her unique skill. Please do keep sharing your knowledge.

Have a conscious day!

Filip De Pessemier
Founding partner @Begrip.be
Moving People to Solution State
Founder of the Life Improvement Boot Camp

PREFACE

"Tick tock, tick tock, tick tock.... Tick... tock... T...I...C...K T...O... C...K It is 6 o'clock.

My heart is pounding; my breathing is erratic... I am getting confused and I feel my chest is compressed in a knot...

Tick tock, tick tock, tick tock, it is 6 o'clock, I can hear the steps on the stairs, getting closer and closer, the key in the key hole turning like a knife in my gut, tic toc it is 6 o'clock... Last breath in..."

I was giving one of my presentations to my colleagues. They were enthralled by me, they were in my story, they could feel the steps on the stairs, they could feel my heart pounding. I was feeling so excited to be able to make a picture with my words.

I was at the Public Speakers University. A very intense course created by Andy Harrington. Andy is a worldwide successful public motivational speaker who has designed a multi layered programme to make you a confident and successful speaker.

It is so amazing to see how momentums in life can trigger a series of events that can change your life.

I found myself following obediently the steps that destiny had put on my path. Everything started very mundane in Facebook. I rarely pay attention to the hundreds of bombarding advertisements of self-improvement courses. How much can you cope with people telling you they have the answer for you to become richer, cleverer, happier.

This time I felt I was driven to attend to one of Andy's free talks. I knew that nothing is for free that it is the tendency now to offer lots of free information and present it in such a way to make you to buy. That it is the savvy and cynical side of myself who has survived in a jungle of clever advertisement and marketing based on psychological behaviour studies and Neuro Linguistic Programming (NLP) and other sciences where they observe us like monkeys in a cage to find the better way to squeeze us from our last penny.

I was compelled to follow as I felt this was my moment to trigger a change in my life. I have learnt through experience to identify these moments and to act and jump into the opportunity despite not knowing what I was getting into.

And then, there she was, this brunette who looked like a Hawk. She owned the stage like a bird of prey flying left to right and centre. Cheryl was so majestic, putting soul in each word, a master in action, so powerful, so viscerally female despite all the swearing that, by the way, sounded so charming in her lips.

PART 1

A life experience

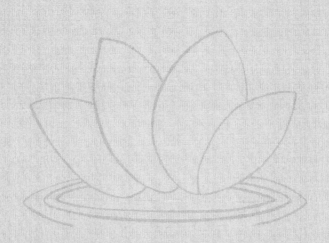

New text message arrived:

"Adriana, I went to watch the Dr. Strange movie and I found it amazing… Great confusing movie but a little bit like you, it is all about what you teach.

I thought of you when I saw the Ancient one, it was like being with you"

I replied: "Thank you I know I am an old woman but Ancient, lol… I hope not"

"Do not be silly" "It is not the age it is you! Your wisdom, your attitude, your characteristics"

They were the messages from Anabel who is one of my clients. I have treated her for several years.

And that it is one of the hundreds of testimonials that I have from my clients.

I realised my purpose in life, that it is helping others, guiding them through a healing process. I have several labels but in short I am a complementary therapist, a healer and a mentor to those who need guidance.

I believe in the ability that we all should heal our own selves. We need sometimes someone, or something that will point us towards creating a bigger understanding and act in the present, in the now where we can give us the chance to develop love, compassion, empathy for our own self.

I love my life, I love myself and when I look back into my life, there is nothing that I would change or regret.

It has been a wonderful experience to whom I have a deep gratitude and the sense of accomplishment and self-realization.

It all started in 1966, in Colombia where I was born.

When I was born, my mother said: "Nena cuando naciste tenias unos ojos marrones muy grandes y mirabas todo…" Sorry mother does not speak English.

What she said was that when I was born I had very big brown eyes and I had a peripheral vision, observing everything and looking deeply into the world like feeling the world in the soul.

A few years later, my father who was a maverick, free spirited pilot, loved farming although he did not have a clue what he was doing.

At the time, I was around 3 years old, we had a cotton farm in Aguachica, In the region of the Cesar in Colombia. It is one of the hottest tropical areas you can imagine, where the heat stops the passing of time, a heat wave that was almost visual, emanating from the ground in desperation to get a breath of fresh air.

There was a river crossing the property where my two older brothers used to play. Mother was pregnant with my younger brother. She spent her time inside of the farmhouse where we used to spend holidays. She was not happy leaving her comfortable house in the city of Bucaramanga.

One day my brothers who were 10 and 8 years old decided to put me in an inflatable pneumatic from an old truck tire and they abandoned me in the river. The current took me away from the house farm, from the land. A fisherman rescued me from the waters and took me back home a few hours later.

I do remember still, the sensation of being in the water, I felt there an energy, a presence looking after me. I did not feel fear nor did I cry. I have images of the water, me floating on it, the voice of the running waters the sensation of being nursed in the arms of a soft maternal Earth.

It has not been the first time I had felt that guardian loving angel around me and taking care of me.

A few months later my parents divorced. We left our home and were forced to go and live with my paternal grandmother in Bogota. Grandmother was a big matron, a giant of 4 feet 5", so strong and the queen mother of the family. She was a wonderful lady but not very keen on girls and she made sure I could experience her feelings from early age.

She was a Machiavellian practitioner, a clever and expert politician. I loved her but we did not share the same principles.

My mother started working in a multinational company and was getting very good at her work and travelling a lot. She had found her calling. She was born to be an executive, a leader, workaholic for whom the idea of motherhood of 4 children was below her competence.

My grandmother's house was an old house. I loved it but it was a house with very strong energy.

My grandfather had died many years ago, he was an artist painter, he studied arts in New York and in the twenties during the USA depression he went back to Colombia. He was very avant-garde for his time. A socialist artist, anti-American, anti-establishment and against oppression of the poor, living in a very conservatism right government.

My grandfather was on the black list of artists who were forbidden to exhibit. He went to jail for exhibiting shocking socialist anti-government paintings.

For a living, he was a cartoonist for The Times in Colombia and he was working as a cartographer at the local geographic institute "Agustin Codazzi".

But my grandfather was also a spiritual man. He was deeply into meditation, a gnostic, vegetarian who built his studio next to the main house where he moved. He spent his time in meditation, spiritual growth and painting when he was not at work.

He was deeply misunderstood and labelled as an eccentric artist into weird things. He died in the early sixties long before I was born.

A lot of strange things happened at that house. We used to have a very old maid who lived at the house for decades. Rufina had grey hair and was so short, full of wrinkles and with a kind look of servitude in her eyes.

On one occasion, she woke up in the middle of the night, screaming and alerting everyone. She told us that she was dreaming and a voice woke her up asking her to stand up right there and to hurry. As soon she moved out of her bed the plaster of the ceiling fell down on top of her bed.

She was more afraid of the voice that saved her life than of the possibility of being underneath a block of concrete.

In another story before my time, my grandparents received a visit from a local priest who was fond of my grandmother. The church of Santa Teresita was around the corner.

The priest had coffee with my grandparents and spent a good hour with them.

A couple of days later they met another priest and mentioned the visit of the other priest. The father told them they may have had the wrong date as that priest died the day before he came to visit them.

It was at that house my psychic experiences starting to become real. I had few episodes at that place.

The most distinct one was the noise. It was when I started hearing vibrations. It was like a blip, a persistent one. When I was closing my eyes, I could see it as a line moving in different directions that was more intense in the corridor above the central patio.

Sometimes, I was having what I could describe as out of body experiences. I was by then 8 years old. It was at night time in bed, I was holding the edges of the bed, feeling like a vortex opening underneath my body, a void pulling me. The energy was so strong, that I was feeling I was above my body and I could see underneath the engulfing vortex with my body vibrating. I was holding the edge of the bed in pure panic to avoid falling into the darkness. It was a such negative energy, so scary.

Voices were talking to me at the same time, I felt like they were trying to drain me, trying to hold me.

I never said anything of my nocturnal terrors to anyone. I just mentioned to mama that I did not like human dolls as they scared me.

A few maids later after our beloved Rufina finally rested in peace, I remembered a new one who was burning herbs. I think it was Sage because to her the house was haunted and bad spirits dwelled there. The herbs were intended to purify the energy.

Funnily enough, she was burning the pot of herbs in the middle of the night in the centre of the patio. The patio where I used to hear that cacophony of blips and lines and wailing voices.

I remember my grandmother waking up and the commotion in the middle of the night accusing the maid of being a witch, an evil demonic witch and fired her on the spot. The woman was out of the house at first light. Fired for witchcraft.

The maid was hysterical and screaming that the house was haunted, that the devil was living there and she was cleaning it.

I was then even more scared than ever. So, I never said anything about my own experiences.

We moved homes when I was 11 to a brand new one. Grandmother stayed at her big house and we started a new life.

I studied at a catholic private only girls' school, Esclavas del Sagrado Corazon de Jesus (Slaves of the Sacred Heart of Jesus). I loved it. I thought that will be my vocation, becoming a nun. My love for the nuns and mainly my love for Jesus was growing every day. I was not really popular or had many friends.

I loved going to spiritual retreats and convents where I felt it was my place.

The nuns provided the first platform for me to feel Jesus. After them, the real church was in our hearts as Jesus lived there. The only thing we had to do was to feel unconditional love and have compassion and be humble. These were attributes that I could relate to.

My favourite place to spend during lunch time at school was at a small chapel, so quiet and all for myself as it seemed I was the only teenager who enjoyed having her breaks in prayer.

In the meantime, at home, also I was seeking the solitude of my room, feeling all these energies and dialogues with God. I was feeling different vibrations; I was getting quite psychic with a few premonitions but my real passion was healing.

I was going around the neighbourhood, which was a relatively new one with many green areas where I found strayed injured or malnourished abandoned dogs and any other animals that I used to nurse at home.

I was looking after them at home until they were getting better. I noticed that with my touch they were healing faster and they felt loved and comforted.

People too were asking me to give them a little massage. My uncle Roberto, used to asked me to touch his head as he had a headache and a lot of stress. He always said I had little healing hands.

I remember an episode when I was 14 years old. A young man was bitten on the face by his dog. The bite was very bad and he had to have plastic surgery. His nose and upper lip were the most affected by the bite. The nose was hanging from a thread of flesh and the upper lip was completely split up and leaving a gap.

His mother called me out of the blue as she knew I was the right person to help to clean his wounds.

He had all the stitches and lots of coagulated blood all over but it was vital to keep the wound free of infection. Without any training and at 14, I felt like I was an expert. I started cleaning the wounds with such confidence as I was an expert. He felt such a relief, he was so grateful and saying that my touch was making him feel so good completely free of pain.

However, I was labelled as a weird girl. My mother struggled to understand that I was so different to other girls of my age. I was not into boys even though they were literally queuing in front of my front door to date me. I was not into fashion, nor shopping, or make-up.

Latin-American culture portrays a very feminine image of girls, even more so when the girl is physically attractive. I never paid attention to this.

I never considered myself to be pretty. It was not in my psyche. I was into reading a lot, mainly philosophy and mystic books. My friends were Socrates, Plato, Kierkegaard and even the poor Nietzsche.

I loved Mythology, arts and biology.

My behaviour was causing issues as I felt no one could understand me. My mother was paying for psychological therapies which were not going anywhere.

At school, as well, they made tests where I came out with a diagnosis of amorphous personality, a shapeless, nebulous, unformed being but intelligent enough to apply to any university.

I had more therapies and I became intellectually knowledgeable of human behaviour such as defence mechanisms, the ego, super ego and object...

Mother became more frustrated as her only daughter was the last being she could identify with. She was an executive for Yardley, the English company for beauty products where glamour and fashion was the order of the day while her daughter was quoting Antoine de Saint Exupery and its Petit Prince, saying "that the real beauty was invisible to the naked eye".

I finished my baccalaureate when I was 16, ahead of the other girls as I did not do year 1 in primary school as I was too bright and I seemed to know all the curriculum of year 1. So, I did one month of year one then I was catapulted to a year ahead. Perhaps my intellect was working but I could not understand the appeal of being a teenager. I thought boys were a nuisance. I went out with a few, but some of them dumped me because I did not want to have sex with them.

To me clothes were practical to cover my body from the cold. I was happy to go to my mother wardrobe and wear something of hers although she was 30 years above my age.

I loved to spend time with the maids and to teach them to read. I remember one of them who I thought she must be dyslexic. I spent days and days trying to explain mechanical clocks to no avail. At the end, I gave her a digital clock!

One of the most humbling beautiful experiences was going with Maria Ines, who was our live-in maid for several years, to visit her family for a weekend.

We left very early to get a coach and we travelled for several hours. We arrived at a small village and then we walked for a couple of hours up hill to a mountain. On top of a hill I saw a small shaky dilapidated hut. We could see the smoke coming out from the left area of the hut, the sun was bright and high and the fresh mountain air was cold. It felt like needles on your face as soon you started accelerating your pace.

When we approached, there were a band of happy laughing red young cheeks coming to greet us. These young children had such happy faces. They were 4 of them and then the mother came with a little girl in her arms with a dirty face with soil covering her red plump cheeks that characterised the tan of the cold mountains.

There was so much love and joy to see their older sister, the provider for the whole family. They were honoured to meet me, the person who just by her presence made them feel ashamed of their poverty.

The hut did not have a floor, they were cooking in a live fire in the left corner of the house. There was only a big bedroom with two double beds, no toilets, nor running water.

Their father has left long ago leaving them at the mercy of the mountain.

For food, they were boiling potatoes. We brought a lot of gifts and sweets for the children that I bought with my pocket money that for them seemed to be a fortune.

They had a couple of hens with little chicks. The mother wanted to kill one of the hens to provide a decent meal for their special guest but I refused categorically because it would break my heart not only to take their food but to kill an innocent animal for my benefit.

I told them that I would be much happier to have the potatoes with an egg if they had any.

We ate, we walked in the mountains and we rested at the edge of a cliff. It was so beautiful, so much harmony and peace. I felt again the presence of God and unconditional love filled my heart again. I felt alive and so overwhelmed with joy and beauty. I was witnessing the invisible beauty and I was so privileged.

I knew my reality was very different to theirs and these conditions could be charming for a weekend but I did not have to walk hours to go to a local school that the sister was paying for or carry water canteens from the local stream.

I honestly felt so happy for them and I hoped I gave them a reason to feel themselves proud of what they were and not impressed by the money and the status I represented.

My race towards being myself and fitting in what my social group was expecting from me was against me. I arrived at the conclusion that I had to lose myself to become someone for them.

My conversations with God, my long hours of meditation, my energy sensitivity and my search for the soul had to be put in hold. They were my guilty pleasures that no one knew about.

I was getting so tired of being judged and considered the black sheep in the family.

Then, the usual path was in front of me. University was there. There was no other option and even I could not choose what was closer to what I wanted, Philosophy and theology, as my mother wanted me to become a dentist.

When I told the family, I wanted to be a nun they refused my option. Father said he would do everything to keep his only daughter outside of the convent. Also, no Philosophy as I will not be able to make a living from it and he would not pay a very expensive private University if he would have to support me after graduation or until I get married to someone who belonged to the same sphere.

Then I started going from university to university. I did a pre-medicine school, then I studied two years of Microbiology at the Andes, which is one of the most privileged universities of the country where only the elite of the intellectuals can attend like going to a Cambridge, or a Harvard.

After two years of misery and trying to manoeuvring my father to pay for a new university, he refused and told me to take a gap semester and find what to do with my life.

By then, I had met one of my best friends, at the Andes University. I had a very eclectic group of friends from the nerdiest ones, such as biologists and scientists with whom I was enjoying trips to nature and study lichens and crocodiles to textile designers and artists.

Liliana was one of my designer friends. She was amazing. A few years older than me, she was so bohemian and free spirited. What my mother was asking me to do in previous years I started to do by then. I was going to exquisite and strange decadent parties. They were misfits, models, artists, architects, designers, bohemian thinkers. I realised that I could be an observer. They knew I had a different energy. I have never been into drugs and I was not going to start then. I was not into drinking either but they accepted me. I was most probably the youngest of them all.

I was treated with respect and affection. I was admired for myself, not being judged and they cared for me, protected me. My mother was horrified as she could not see the deeper picture.

Then I went back to university as time ran out and Liliana suggested fashion design as I had to apply for something. As the fees were for a design school at a fraction of the Andes my father was happy to pay.

I got tired and I started feeling that emptiness again. I felt spiritual calls again but I was consciously fighting them.

As usual I was academically gifted but the energy was getting stagnant and putrid.

I was dating someone much older than me, over 15 years older. This was a very interesting period when I learnt so much. This man was a very influential man, powerful and decadent at the same time.

He was involved with the peace process with a national guerrilla group called   the M19.

They were a band of terrorists mixed up in drugs trafficking and extortion. There were secret meetings with Ambassadors, politicians, ex-presidents and I was there in the shadows. I was the adviser of the adviser, the support and moral compass behind the curtains.

This man I dated was into drugs and alcohol and I was his little twinkle bell.

They were such decadent people. Lots of them thieves and criminals even killers, they became a seductive magnet to the boyfriend. A blanket of dark shadows covered our relationship.

I became the only source of light used as a shield to bring sanity to this man.

In the meantime, one day at Liliana's house, on an Easter Friday, a group of her friends were playing with a Ouija board.

I never liked those sort of things, but I arrived when they were playing it.

As soon I got closer to them they left and I found myself alone with it. I touched it and the pointer started to move by itself.

Then I felt different. Something got inside of me. I felt as I felt many years ago, at my grandmother's house that pressure of that sound that scared me so much when I was a child.

I felt suicidal but at the same time it was not my feeling, it was like I was not alone inside of myself.

I told Liliana what happened and she was very scared. Her mum and her aunt who lived at the house came to pray for me. We went to the local Catholic church and the priest dismissed the episode. He thought we were suggestable girls.

We went back to her house as I told her I could not be alone or drive back to my home as I was seeing in my mind crutching my car on purpose. At her house, I started telling them things that happened in their house a long time before I met them, I also pointed to antiques that were holding negative energies. These were objects that were already "cleaned" by a medium in previous visits.

Liliana and I shared her bed that night. In her room, she used to have on top of her bed a Japanese sabre.

In the middle of the night I screamed and sat up in the bed pulling Liliana towards me telling her to sit up. At that moment that sabre felt pointing downwards into the pillow where we were sleeping. We were petrified with fear. My eyes looked different.

The next morning, we went to a clairvoyant psychic medium that the family knew very well.

Nina Lozano de Afanador was her name. A very old lady, short and round, who reminded me of my grandmother. As soon she opened the door of her house she knew what happened. She knew I was the object of the enquiry and she held me. She made a ritual on my back and I started feeling more myself. She told me that I was a very special being, full of light, that I came to this world to do a lot of good but I attracted a desperate soul. This was a young man who killed himself who could not pass over and he was attracted to my energy.

She gave us the name and the place of the cemetery where he was buried. It was real.

From then she took me under her wing. I became her driver taking her to visit all these rich families that were using her services. I did not like that. I did not want to be a clairvoyant myself. We had a lovely relationship and she introduced me into a mystical world.

I got involved with gnostic people and again I found myself at the centre of their group as they were using me to connect with high energies. I witnessed Saint Michael archangel several times coming through me.

I was going to well-known churches like the 20 de Julio church, to visit the little Jesus, that had been accredited with so many miracles. I started to feel these energies again so strongly even more intense than ever. My only love was God and Jesus. The frantic fervent desire to become one with God was more and more intense.

By now the boyfriend was using me like a token of good energy. Taking me to his meetings to see what I felt about X or Y person. He was asking me to predict if his new business ventures would go ahead or asking me for protection.

The so-called friends were just interested in me telling them events of their past or what could I "see".

In one episode while visiting the group of Gnostics, I got a message. I had broken up my relationship with the boyfriend in several occasions and it was more death than alive.

But I had to do something for him. He was in imminent danger this time. I saw angels at my command going to look after him.

By then he became a very close friend to Pizarro who was the leader of the M19.

I tried to call him and I left him a message to warn him about the danger but he never answered the phone. I started to feel the familiar heavy confusing energy from the past.

I prayed and asked God to protect him. A few hours later it was in the news. Pizarro was on a plane which was going to a provincial city on the Caribbean Colombian coast, (my ex-boyfriend was supposed to go with him and seated next to him), when someone who was sitting in the row behind him took a gun and killed Pizarro with a bullet in the head.

I could not contact my ex-boyfriend so I did not know what happened to him.

Later, he told me that very strange things had happened to him that morning. Nothing went as planned, his driver was late, the car did not work, the traffic was horrendous and he missed his plane.

He took the following plane and he found out what happened when he landed.

After, that my time with him was over. He looked at me with more fear and just as an object to be used for personal gain.

A few years passed and I was finally graduated as a Fashion designer. Again, I had another period of spiritual rejection and silence. The Gnostics were history, the reading of metaphysical teaching was over and my relationship with Nina was gone.

I felt a new call, I had to leave the country. I was in my last year preparing my thesis for university. I had had a few broken relationships and Liliana was out of the picture.

I had a very bad relationship with mother as she was poisoned against me by my hideous sister in law. That woman was a gold digger and she knew I could see through her from day one.

The sister- in-law was shamefully skilled in squeezing money from my family and no one could see her lies and trickery. My mother finally admitted that for years I was right and that she was not the person she thought she was. Mother even told me that the ill treatment I was victim of was because of all the lies she created. She even told the whole family that I was a lesbian and I tried to seduce her…

As if, I told mama I was not attracted to ladies but even if it was the case my sister in law was not my type.

The situation in the country was getting worse with Pablo Escobar on the loose and there was a wave of terrorism. Again, the same oppressing energy from my childhood. I was so unhappy.

The call of moving abroad came a reality in 1990. I found myself at the mercy of the Universe that took me to Paris. Everything went so smoothly as designed by a higher intelligence. I arrived in Paris flying in first class, after running away from home with the father's promise that I would never get a penny from him if I left the country!

How beautiful is the Universe working in synchronicity, that gave me the chance to say good bye to my grandmother who died a couple of days before my flight. My father and his family, and my mother and her husband came to say good bye at the airport. My beloved younger brother was my accomplice and he to this today has all my love and gratitude.

I got married for the first time to a young sweet gorgeous angel. I felt God sent him to look after me.

I spent 6 years in Paris. I found myself studying again, the eternal student, fashion again, that I really hated. Then I studied at the Sorbonne, French and French civilisation followed by International trade management at the Ecole Normale Superieure de Cachan.

By then I felt another spiritual call. I found myself visiting a few churches where I found the energy was very strong. I was becoming a recluse and feeling the psychic connection again.

However, my young husband who was from a traditional Catholic family was quite scared of all this bewitchment so again I found myself living a double life and miserable.

We were growing apart and I was now a woman and no longer a young girl.

Again, I felt that France was not my destination. Another call, another synchronicity, took me to London.

I arrived in London without having anywhere to live and I felt like as I did in that river over 25 years ago.

I sensed a force was looking after me. I finally realised that I had arrived where I needed to be. England was home.

Despite finding myself in difficult situations I ended up living in Shalcomb Street in Chelsea at a house of a very eccentric lady who rented rooms to students.

I had amicably divorced my ex-husband with the same lawyer and with no alimony as it was after all me who left him. I said to him that because my love for him was unconditional and I was full of gratitude I had to leave him free to find the woman who would love him and with whom he could be really happy. We were not happy during the previous two years and it was time for us to be free.

One year later he was living in the South of France with a new job and a new partner. I was so happy for him.

I found myself studying again. This time I was studying English at Westminster College.

I was going to a church in Chelsea that funnily enough caught my attention because it had indoor fences. I went to meditate and pray, recalling my lunchtimes at school. By now, the feeling of emptiness was getting stronger and stronger. I was getting more introverted. Sometimes, I spent several days without talking to anybody. I just dedicated my time to pray and meditate.

It was the only time that I felt happy and able to understand the world.

I had made a handful of friends in Chelsea, one of whom was my dearest friend Irving Press. He was my second "Liliana" representing the opposite that I was. He was into the glamour and the decadent world in Mayfair and Chelsea. He was the master of ceremonies in the fashionable night clubs, restaurants and parties. What a beautiful sensation, the air of success, the superior feeling when you entered a club without the need to join a queue! The funny thing was that I became an observant of this world where no one really bothered me.

Then in 1998 I got married to a banker who was working in the City and we were living in a charming flat in SW3, in the heart of Chelsea.

In 1999 our beautiful baby boy, our Drew, was born.

My husband was a very charming tall blonde handsome American man. A New Yorker with the looks of a younger Clint Eastwood. He was in his late forties so there was a considerable difference in age that provided reassurance and stability.

His mother was a wonderful lady. Born and raised in Long Island and married to another banker and living in Manhattan. She divorced many years ago, and my father in law died long before I met him. Barbara remarried to a wonderful man, a widower father of five and she raised them as hers.

When I met my mother in-law she used to live in Palm Beach in Florida and, she had a second residency in Long Island, a charming little cabin in the beach for her Summer times as Florida was too hot. My husband spent his younger years in the Jesuit school in Manhattan then studies in Anthropology and master degrees in Business.

He was a remarkable intelligent man able to seduce you with a clever remark. He was so well travelled, he had worked around the globe!

My mother was so happy finally, her daughter made it. Finally, she could tell her friends and relatives that her damaged daughter was not a loser after all.

But there was a secret. My banker was a functioning addict. He was addicted to drugs; marihuana, cocaine, alcohol, women, cigarettes… any way it seemed to be addicted to everything but mainly he was addicted to cruelty. His addiction to hurt me was perhaps the worst of all.

He was Doctor Jekyll and Mr. Hyde. The most erratic behaviour changing so fast, becoming suddenly so aggressive, cruel and violent particularly during the pregnancy. He did unspeakable things to me during the pregnancy that took me deeper into the field of the darts of existence.

My pregnancy was a blanket of fear and sadness, I tried so hard to protect my sweet baby. I was talking to him as I felt his presence and his love was giving me hope and that everything would be fine. My baby saved my life as he was my source of love and light giving me the strength to carry on in love with life despite the abuse.

Dark and fearful times, once, when I was six months pregnant, we were in Antibes, visiting one of his friends. Duncan was a social parasite, with no skills neither a job. Duncan had a house in Belgravia, his mother got permanent social housing for years and he "inherited" her house. It was a three-bedroom house with a very big garden, humble but spacious and with character. He rented the rooms in the house and claimed unemployment benefits. This allowed him to have a second residence where he spent mostly of his time in Antibes in the French Riviera living with his partner who could not be much older than the half of his age.

The flat in Antibes was in the heart of the old town, in the main plaza, mediaeval houses converted into small charming little flats, just a few yards away from the harbour and market.

Duncan and my husband were the best of friends, high on drugs every time they were together. One evening the three of them went out and I went to bed. In the middle of the night my husband pulled me out of the bed by my hair. He was hitting me and dragged me to the kitchen floor.

He kicked me and shouted: YOU ARE TAKING ALL THE SPACE IN THE BED BITCH! You and your fat tummy bloody FU*** C***. You are going to sleep on the kitchen floor as I am getting the bed for myself, DID YOU HEAR ME?

When he left, I took some kitchen towels and I made a nest for myself to lie on, but he saw it and came at me again. He pulled the towels underneath my body and I was rolling on the floor. He was screaming at me, telling me: "You do not have the right to put anything on the floor, I told you to sleep on the floor like the animal that you are…" I screamed asking for help in English and in French, A l'aide, a l'aide! I called Duncan and his girlfriend but no one came, no one helped.

I was just there lying on the floor in a foetal position protecting my belly, staring underneath the cooker looking at all the dirt. I even saw my husband's wedding ring who in his anger threw it to my face and it landed underneath the cooker. I was just there, just thinking of that dirt underneath, how filthy it was and I smiled saying to myself at least I do not have to clean this place.

No one came, the sun rose and I was there on the floor with dried tears on my face knowing that I was all alone and that I had to protect my baby myself and I had to do that alone. There was no point asking for help as no one was bothered.

How low I felt, how decadent was his world. His friends were an abomination, so noxious and corrupted. The hypocrisy, the double standards, the selfishness, dirty weak souls. I was the only pure and clean thing in his life, like a delicate flower with an intense innocent beauty in a world of thorns, putrefying darkness, twisted vines, fermented thistles of weakness and fakery.

You could see them on the surface with the big positions, high executives of Investment banks. One of them was so infamous, with all his proper and perfect life. With a wife of leisure, just concerned in fitting in with her rich girlfriends. She spent her hours trying to impress with fancy luncheons at her house for the Chelsea Flower Show as they lived literally at the corner of the Royal Hospital Road.

Double standards characterised this people. He used my husband to avoid to get his hands dirty. Every time he wanted cocaine and party he called my husband to contact the dealer. Their cocaine dealer was such a disgusting man, short, bold, fat and greasy, with short fingers, repulsive and greedy. My husband's friend knew he was an addict. He also knew my husband had been in rehab several times, and he criticised him behind his back and pointed with a moralising finger. He was washing his hands saying he tried to help him like a Pontius Pilatus crucifying a poor devil. How little weight good intentional friendship had when his desire to have a line of cocaine made him forget his good intentions as after all his consumption was only "recreational".

Their dinner parties were funny, we were rarely invited as we were not up to their standards; it seemed our presence was appreciated only when they wanted a buffoon to get the drugs for them. I think I was the only one eating and enjoying the food on their table, as all of them were high on cocaine and no one else was eating.

I several times questioned him and his wife who was my so-called friend. I asked what type of friendship is the one that knowingly your friend is an addict you ask him to get drugs for your amusement and totally careless of the wellbeing of your friend and his family?

How can you criticise my husband and say how shameful his behaviour is, and how sad and go on and on, when he was one of the instigators for his selfish recreation? This guy several times was asking me for Barbara. She was one of my friends who I met with Irving. She was a beautiful Brazilian model/actress who was cast in the Bond movies.

I found this a little bit puzzling as I never introduced her to the friend. He was constantly asking after her with a ridiculous nervous laugh like they were having a private joke at my expense.

Later, Irving told me he had confronted my ex-husband several times and got into a fight with him as Barbara contacted Irving asking him for help as my husband was harassing her, calling her and not leaving her alone. My husband got her contact details from my personal contact list and tried to seduce her. And that was the joke!

Irving was my saviour so many times, he intervened and protected me from my husband. I ended staying at his house for days during my pregnancy when my husband was out of control.

All that atmosphere was so unhealthy, you can see their intentions and their lies and fake. Young women throwing themselves to rich guys just with the hope of getting a financial gain, crumbs and small tokens reduced sometimes just to a few lines of cocaine.

They got impressed by their titles and careers, their well-travelled experiences and fancy addresses but they could not see the cynicism and corrupted hearts, the cheating and the twisted darkness.

There was one of them who was a dentist. A Harley street dentist! What a laughing matter. The guy was such a cocaine addict that he shared his practice with my husband's fatty cocaine dealer. He had his private office at the dentist, a perfect cover. One night my husband got a dental emergency, in the middle of the night, he called his pal and we ended up at his practice. These two guys were both so high that he treated the wrong tooth. He made a root canal in the wrong tooth! I had to take my husband the next day to the hospital.

The day my boy was born was probably one of the worse, as I started labour by midnight and that man literally kicked me out of my bed as

I was making too much noise and he could not sleep. I prepared a hot bath to reduce the pain and at every contraction I was biting my knuckles to reduce the noise but with little success, as he came to the bath and threatened to punch me in the face, his closed fist against my eye, if I carried out making noise.

I was checking my own contractions and getting out the bath. I used the phone in living room to call the hospital. By 4 am they told me to go to the hospital. I told them I did not have a car so they suggested to me to call an ambulance. When I was dialling 999, he came behind me and started to shout ordering me to hang up. Luckily for me the gentleman on the other side of the line was listening and he told me to ignore him and that he would send the ambulance and if necessary the police as well.

He told me to stay on the phone until the ambulance arrived! My husband was arguing that it was very embarrassing to have an ambulance in the front of the building, what would the neighbours think! He wanted me to get dressed and go to the street and get a taxi instead.

When the paramedics arrived, he was Mr Kind, telling them how grateful he was to them for coming to pick US up! He was hugging me and telling them that I was his precious wife and he could not wait for our baby to be born!

I stayed in the Chelsea and Westminster Hospital for 3 days despite that it was a normal birth. I had a few small complications and being asthmatic did not help either but mainly I was so afraid of going home to that man and the doctors knew it. As soon the baby was born, the husband left so I had to go from the labour room to my bed and shower all by myself, carrying baby and bags and with no help, all alone.

The doctors at the third day told me they could not allow me to stay any longer at the hospital. They said they had been very sympathetic so far but they needed the bed. They told me that I had to go back home or going to a Refuge and said: "A young pretty lady like you does not deserve to go to a place like that, you would not like to be in a place like that".

The husband came to pick me up, against hospital policy. He did not bring any car seat for the baby, he just told me: "grab the child and run when I tell you, as I am not going to buy any shit seat". At least he paid for a taxi!

I was so right to be scared. One week later I found myself at Heathrow airport; my little brother had sent me the ticket and I was running from my ex-husband again. A few days before I went to the French consulate to register Drew under my passport and then we were on our way to Boston, seeking refuge at my brother's.

Life was so miserable. It was a living hell with that man. It seemed he could not understand that I was not fit and well enough to be a slave. As he did not allow anyone to help me and he was calling from his office several times a day to make sure the phone was not engaged. I was not talking to anyone, I was completely by myself except for a couple of friends.

The tiredness and the hormones and his demands where so high that I could not cope by myself. I arrived in Boston broken and exhausted. My brother and his partner Larry were such a wonderful help. They were there two guys taking care of the baby. For them Drew was a gift as he was like the child they could not biologically conceive. So many presents, clothes toys!... Wow, it was everything we did not have at home.

I was so depressed and my sadness and fear knowing that sooner or later I had to go back to London to my nightmare. We spent over 4 weeks there and my mother in law and her husband came to pick us up from Long Island. They adored Drew, he was so beautiful and his grandmother was so happy to hold him in her arms. Long island was an oasis of peace, I spent the days in the beach alone with no a soul to see, a gentle end of summer breeze, with wonderful colours, the fields of sunflower were in an explosion of yellow petals, orange and brown seeds. The woods were kind and warm with a hint of brownish autumn colours to come. Pumpkins were growing on the floor looking like columns of an army of terracotta soldiers facing the sea.

Alas my days there were numbered. Barbara my mother in law, had been in peace talks, negotiating my entry to the Chelsea residence. She was imposing her matriarchal power to force her son to be a human being. I stayed in America for 7 weeks. It was time to face the music!

At my arrival in London, he was waiting for us at the airport with a new pariah friend. We had an overnight flight and we arrived early in the morning. My husband and his friend were still high from their drug rampage and they had not slept at all.

When I arrived home, I went to lie down and breastfed the baby. I noticed a new decoration on the wall above the headrest of the bed, it was red nail burnish vertical marks, perhaps as a souvenir of some sexual activity taking place while I was enjoying the sunflower fields.

I was so tired and with jet lag that I just stripped off the bed the dirty sheets and I rested. A few minutes had passed and this guy came like a rhinoceros towards me. He started to insult me and call me names. He said that he was hungry and that the flat had not been cleaned for 2 months. He demanded I stand up and earn my place at home that his mother was not there to tell him what to do or not.

As he saw the baby breastfeeding, he said to me if your excuse for lying like a cow is feeding that thing I will take it away from you, he started throwing towards us everything he found handy; Drew's little cot, baby bags, furniture, pillows... I covered the baby with my body then this man went to the other side of the bed and pulled Drew by the feet with such a force that separated him from my breast and put him at the end of the bed. The baby was crying, scared and upset. I jumped to grab him and took him under my chest while this man was throwing things over my back. By a miracle, I managed to grab the phone and I called the police who were there in minutes.

When he realised I had called the police he ran to hide the drugs he had in the flat.

Two police officers came, one interviewed me in the master bedroom and the other was with him in the living room.

He denied everything but the police noticed he was under the influence of drugs. They asked me and I confirmed it. I told them everything but they did not take any action.

They told me if I called them again, they would have to take me away to a refuge. They said to me to think twice to call them as I was too pretty and proper to survive in a place like that. "That place is not for a lady like you". They told me to think of the baby.

The police told him that if he touched me or the baby they would come back and take him to jail.

Their visit made things worse as he became even more psychologically cruel. He was threating me with his fist just stopping a few millimetres away from my eye, saying to me he would not give me the satisfaction to see him in jail and I would never get a witness to his behaviour so it was my word against his.

Tick tock, tick tock, tick, tock, it is 6 o'clock.

Tick Tock, TICK TOCK, TICK TOCK. Tick tock... my heart is pounding again this node in my gut, I am getting nervous and confused. I do not know what to do... Six o'clock, I can hear his walk in the street. He has stopped in front of the building, he just entered, he is downstairs, I am breathing heavily, my asthma is flaring up.

He is here, he is here. I am like a euphoric ant, double checking everything as he demands perfection depending on the mood of the day. His standard of measuring quality could be very draconian. Most probably the temper would be a dark one as he has not taken any drugs for the past 10 hours. So, the first thing would be going for his marihuana that stinks so badly after of course insulting me…

I can hear his steps one after another then the key in the keyhole turning around, then the door opened and slam…

"WHERE IS MY DINNER, WHY IS NOT ON THE TABLE, YOU KNOW THAT AS SOON YOU HEARD ME CLIMBING THE STAIRS IS THE SIGN FOR YOU TO PUT THE FOOD ON THE TABLE AS I DO NOT LIKE MY FOOD COLD OR WAIT FOR YOU TO SERVE IT"

Shouting in my ear, and then "why is the bloody baby here, I cannot relax with the kid here, take him into his room" "Go to breathe somewhere else you taking my air in the same room annoys me, GET OUT of here!"

"YOU ARE NOTHING, DO YOU HEAR ME, YOU ARE NOTHING, YOU DO NOT HAVE A SAY HERE MUTE YOU ARE HERE A SLAVE TO CLEAN AND COOK, YOU CANNOT SAY ANYTHING AS MONEY TALKS AND I AM THE MONEY HERE" If I bring women here (as I found an used condom in my bedroom and I made the mistake to ask him how he dared to disrespect my house like that) YOU DO NOT HAVE the right to say anything as you are less than nothing. You will clean the bed instead!

The mental and emotional abuse was so cruel. I was a trophy abused wife. On the surface was the perfect family a banker living in Chelsea with a young, pretty, well-educated wife and a gorgeous healthy baby boy.

He was so controlling, isolating me from relatives and friends. Several times he insulted my friends and asked them to leave his house when they were visiting me. I could not speak Spanish at home as he needed to understand everything I said and he did not allow my mother or his to come for the birth of my child.

At the entrance to the flat, there was a lean, elegant table. On it, we had some decorations. In the middle of the table was a china bowl, a white porcelain small sized bowl with some Chinese blue arabesques. My husband very creatively named the begging bowl. Every time he was putting small change, not even £1 coins, that begging bowl was what I had access to. "You can only take money from here if you need to buy water for the baby when you take him to the park. This is not for you, if you are getting hungry in the street, you come and eat here. If you get thirsty you come back home and get some tap water, DO YOU HEAR ME? THE BEGGING BOWL IS YOURS, as it is the only thing you deserve, beggar. Remember you are here to clean, cook and take care of the child"

During the whole pregnancy, he never contributed to any expenses, the few maternity clothes I got and Drew's pushchair and all the baby clothes, toys, blankets, were sent by my mother and my little brother from Boston in America. That was one of his conditions to allow me to carry on with the pregnancy as he wanted me to abort my baby. He agreed to have us at home only if he did not have to pay for anything. Even my son's Christening party where all his friends were invited was paid with my savings.

He was doing the food shopping, mainly the price reduced groceries as they were slightly damaged or on the last day of the recommended date while he was wearing Hermes and Cartier.

He was getting worse and worse, not coming home for days and when he finally arrived he was so ill, so intoxicated that his body was soaking wet in sweats and shivering feeling that this time he was going to die of an overdose. In his way down from the drugs, he was so dangerous like a trapped wild animal.

The attacks of profound anger and violence then periods of depression and shame and regrets for all the damaged that his guilty conscious could bare.

Someone is knocking on the door. I opened and a soft kind voice says to me:" Are you ready? Cover yourself and the baby very well as it is cold outside. Do you have everything that you need?"

She was a lovely sweet lady. A little bit shorter than me in the chunky side. She handled a bag with gifts for me and Drew.

She was a Chelsea Social worker who picked me up at home to drive me to a Refuge for Victims of domestic violence.

It was the 21st of December 2000, winter time with a Christmassy atmosphere. There were decorations in Kings road and in Peter Jones around the corner, people were all over like busy bees collecting nectar.

My Chelsea days were over, I was going to Chiswick. My Chelsea friends also departed, only Irving and another couple stayed faithful.

I opened a bag of gifts, toiletries, two Violet Melchett (name of the centre in Chelsea for Social services) T-shirt and jumper, some new underwear, and chocolates and toys for Drew.

My baby, coat, handbag and my gift bag were my only possessions when I arrived to the Refuge. Right there in front of us there was an old Edwardian house, a 4-storey house, with a big red door.

That would be my home from now on, the house with the red door.

I felt on top of the mountain, my Everest, courageous and so strong; I had left! It was over and I was not afraid anymore. Alas, as soon the door was opened, my hopes went down my hills.

A wave of stench, a mixture of an enclosed airless space mixed with dirty nappies and the smell of spitted formula that time forgot to clean from the carpets. There was a cacophony of different cooking with a palette of different tones of smells of fresh and old. The noise of children crying, screaming, loud televisions. An over enthusiastic little girl holding your hand and calling for your attention asking very impertinent questions.

You could not even see what colour the walls were. The dirt; the characteristic little and bigger dirty palm hands in brown dark colour marked a light wall that reminding me of the chiaroscuro of cave paintings from a prehistoric era.

The floors were in an even more pitiful state than the walls. At the entrance, you had to overcome a series of obstacles like in a hurdle jumping competition full of pushchairs.

The Chelsea Social worker was in tears holding my hand. Oh, my God she muttered. I am so sorry to bring you here.

The key workers were so kind. It was like going back to that invisible beauty in the hut in the mountains.

I expected to see red plump winter cheeks while mounting the stairs to the top floor where my room N.6 was waiting for me.

The top floor had clean walls, they were an apple green colour. It had a stair fence to avoid little children going down the stairs so it was my natural barrier towards unwanted visitors from below.

The No. 6 was marked in pen, blue pen, not a marker just some fine repetitive lines contouring the curves of the number six.

My room was a big one. As it was on the top floor it had irregular ceilings and some areas were very low. I liked it.

There were no curtains, a bench bed, two single beds, and old cheap commode that looked like it was a donation that spent several years in total neglect.

I had a sink that I loved. The room had windows one facing the road and the second one facing the fire stairs with a lateral view to a beautiful big garden.

We had a bathroom and toilet opposite our door for the use of rooms 5, 6 and 7. Room 7 was for a single lady and not a family!

The social worker gave me a hug, feeling so guilty for driving me to such a place but again I felt the sensation of floating on the river waters and I said to her "Thank you. We are going to be okay".

The next morning, I bought a cheap round rug that I put in the landing of our floor, I bought a plant that I still have, some cushions and a throw to put in the lounge as it was so insanitary to even dare think about sitting on the sofa.

I was accused of being OCD as I cleaned the walls from the basement where the kitchens were to the top floor were my room was. As I could not stand the idea of my 16-month-old boy getting an infection. I boiled water and used cleaning products and I mopped all the carpets where there was a chance Drew would be.

The first suggestion I made in the house meetings was to create a rota for cleaning the common areas and put areas of not eating or changing nappies as they were social areas and the first point for any new woman coming in.

I did not know what was more shocking, the violence at home or the assault to your dignity at the arrival to this place.

I bought, in a local DIY place, some adhesive metallic numbers that I put in the top floor, 5, 6 and 7.

Finally, looked more like a floor of apartments and not a ghetto with graffiti written numbers in pen on the door.

I spent 26 months there. The first day living there, we were taken to the most humiliating place, to the inquisitionist, the so-called welfare department to make a claim for housing and income support benefits.

What a nightmare, what I was getting into. The scepticism, the patronising attitude, the disregard for your pain and fears. I was not an observer of life any more. Dante's inferno was real. I was not in the boat anymore. I had a short stop and a glance to human misery. My misery.

I was a French citizen, an immigrant with a young little boy, who in their eyes should not be on benefits as my previous address discriminated against me.

The Chelsea label was a heavy cross to carry. I was there because I really had the need. Again, it was like a tick tock tick tock situation, you are nothing again. They have the right to deprive you of any dignity and make you relive the most painful episodes with your husband and the child to prove them that I really was entitled to the benefits.

An inquisitive reluctant eye rose an eyebrow and explained to my key worker that they will provide the benefits, founding myself in Kafkaesque situation.

I felt like an abandoned dog who finally would be entitled to a Kennel in a shelter until permanent housing would be provided.

I spent the most gratifying 26 months of my life at the Refuge. I got time to heal, my 6 o'clock syndrome passed, I was diagnosed with PTSD (Post-Traumatic Stress Disorder). I took advantage of the wonderful psychotherapists who helped me to recover. I became a voice for the Refuge. I was helping the newcomers, young mothers and other single ladies, mainly Muslim ones who were running from their own brothers and fathers.

My life was portrayed in a Christmas appeal on the television programme

"This Morning". It was important to portrayed that violence happens at every level not only against poor immigrant people, and that mental and emotional abuse was as devastating or even more than physical abuse.

I started to study again. I did courses in computing. I studied International Trade Management this time in English at the Institute of Export.

Then suddenly the energy was returning. But this time it was a darker one.

One of the residents told me of a church that they do deliverances, it was the first time that I heard the use of this word meaning to expel and cast out demons.

I went there with her. It was a Catholic church. As soon as the priest approached me a force took over me as when I met Nina. The priest panicked when he saw my reaction, I was twisting, shouting, screaming then I fell on the floor. They took me to the rectory and pinned me down. There were five of them and they could hardly control me.

They sent me to a specialist in London. He was a beautiful corpulent tall man with smooth ebony skin from the Caribbean islands.

He had a flat in East London on a council estate. It was a very cosy one bed room floor. The most important feature was a statue of the Holy Virgin Mary in an altar with candles and other religious paraphernalia.

He saw me for the first time and he knew my nature. He blessed me and said:" You are holy among the holy ones. You are very special lady and you are one of the most beautiful souls I have ever met.

We had so many rituals where again I found myself pinned down and with this man restraining me invoking the holy spirit and Jesus to rescue me from my foes.

Again, terrifying episodes that were draining me of all energy and so painful.

You are having lots of attacks from dark forces; he said. Also, there are lots of souls in pain seeking into your light for a final destination. There are legions of dark soldiers who are stopping you to reach higher levels of self-realisation as you have a great mission and you will become a powerful being bringing light to the darkness. Big battles are awaiting you". And God, he was right. For several years after seeing him, I had so many spiritual encounters with darkness.

Different churches, different experts. The last one that I had the honour to work with was a kind gentle soft man. He was from the island of Grenada, and he was living in Ealing.

He was a man of faith and devoted to serve fellow beings who were in distress. I met him in a Christian Church in Ealing, where I was having deliverance seasons without lot of success if I may say.

I went to their prayer groups as I felt comforted and he was there preaching. We connected straight away. He also could see the force of the Spirit in me. We started working together and he was visiting home for excruciating contortionist sessions of so much pain and release. He was a very tall man, and again, I found so many times twisting and struggling on the floor of my living room and him trying to restrain me.

Foreign voices came out of my throat telling him the same story. "She is precious, she is powerful, she has been sent to cast us out and to bring light in to the world, we cannot let her to do so" He, inspired by our work went to found a church in Grenada.

… Things were improving, all my psychological scars were healing, my life in the Refuge was more or less pleasant. I had fantastic floor mates and we were having such a good time.

But they we rehoused long before me and I stayed there, I was the longest serving resident. I spent more time than any other resident to get a home.

Once was a young Spanish lady living at the Refuge and she had a little boy. Her mother came to visit from Spain so she was staying with her daughter for a few days.

The daughter came and asked me if I could give a massage to her mother. I found the request strange but I went to the room like when I was 14 years old helping people who were in need.

They were on the second floor so they were not part of my floor mates.

I massaged the old lady and she was telling me how good my hands felt that it was like a blessing for her body she felt like healing was going on inside. While I was treating her, I saw lots of confusing colours and lights all over her body.

When I finished, I told her what I had seen and I asked her if she was ill with a chronic disease that was spread all over her body. She started crying and she told me she was HIV positive that a few years ago, she had a blood transfusion and she got contaminated with the virus. I held her in my arms until she calmed down.

Then I got another resident in room N5, she was a young mother with a little girl.

One night around midnight, the night before she was moving out to her house in Richmond, she came in panic to my room. She said she felt there was a ghost in her room. She was asleep and she felt a presence.

I went to her room and yes, I felt a presence too.

I do not know how I knew but I started talking to this presence. I spoke to the young girl and I explained that it was her mother who killed herself.

Her mother also was a victim of domestic violence but she killed herself instead of running away and left her daughter at the mercy of abuse.

Then the daughter has repeated the same story perpetuating domestic abuse.

That soul wanted to make peace and ask for forgiveness. I saw the hand of the mother reaching the daughter's. I told the daughter to extend her hand then she felt her mother's presence. She healed and forgave her and she made peace in tears. She said thank you and forgave her mum and told her she will never allow abuse in her life ever again and the presence left the room.

The girl cried and was so grateful.

The next morning, I got finally my anticipated letter offering my house. It was the only offer. I panicked as I did not know the area of the address, so I looked at an A to Z. I realised that the streets in the area were the names of Saints. The feeling of navigating over the river waters and rescued by the noble fisherman came back and I felt that everything would be again OK.

I arrived at my house in the 13th of February 2003, after living 26 months in the Refuge.

It was winter and the house was empty. The kitchen did not have any appliances.

I became acquainted with Argos while living in the refuge, where one of our best times was getting their catalogues and circling with pen all the things we dreamt of having for our new homes.

I had already saved some money and bought a few things. Money was little as after waiting over a year for my divorce settlement I did not get any alimony. My ex-husband had promised me that I would not get a penny from him and he fulfilled his promise. He hid his money and over spent and was in huge debt. As the judge said to him, he had never seen anything like it. He enjoyed expensive weekends in Montecarlo, Saint Tropez and Antibes. It seems the French Riviera suited him while I was living in a room in a refuge with his child.

The first things I bought were a double sleeping bag and a microwave.

Drew and I slept for a few weeks on the floor in my sleeping bag, the two of us, holding each other. I was so happy!

We were eating food prepared in the microwave, one of the main staples in the house was tin food including Spam meat.

Argos filled my house, with credit card on hand and thanks to a grant and my mother's help who came to visit us in our new home. She bought us a lot of the furniture.

During the time I spent at the refuge, mother and I had serious arguments as she could not believe I left Chelsea to live in a room in a slum. She wanted me to go back to Colombia, and live with her and her husband but I felt it was not my destiny. My inner voice pushed me to be strong and hold my ground in the UK. Perhaps my pride as well, I did not want to go back after a defeat. I would stand up again and even reach higher places no matter if I felt I had to fight the whole world.

The shame on the family, she was speechless with her friends and relatives as she could not talk about my whereabouts as she was again ashamed of me. She told me that I was a very bad mother, that I was not fit to be a mother, who exposed the child to that level of poverty. She asked what future could I offer to my son?

We stopped talking during the time I was at the refuge. I even stopped talking Spanish altogether as again I felt abandoned in a river dealing with life all by myself.

Years later, she understood and asked for my forgiveness. She even compared me to my grandfather, the gnostic one, who was ahead of his time and no one could understand. I felt honoured and relieved to see that the judgement had finally ended.

When I was settled at my new home, again the energies started to play around. I had so many visions and apparitions and the psychic activity. Spirits tormented me at night, talking to me, asking for help. A deep inner battle, feeling lost.

I befriended the local vicar, Father Steve, who was a blessing and a comfort. He was aware of my spiritual battles and I could feel his love and kindness towards me. He knew that I was a spiritual being living a life of suffering, poverty and struggle. I reminded him of Santa Teresa of Avila. For Christmas, he gave me her biography as my Christmas present. What a present. I felt understood I could feel it so much that even I knew what the next page was talking about before turning the page. By then the most difficult period started for me.

I was experiencing a dark night of the soul. I read many years ago, while living in France, The Dark Night by Saint John of the Cross. It had an impact on me then but I realised that this time I was living it. This little poem is part of the work of this mystic Catholic Saint, the Ascent of Mount Carmel.

There are several steps in this night, which are related in successive stanzas. The main idea of the poem is the joyful experience of being guided to God. The only light in this dark night is that which burns in the soul. And that is a guide more certain than the mid-day sun: Aquésta me guiaba, más cierto que la luz del mediodía. This light leads the soul engaged in the mystic journey to divine union.

I had periods of deep darkness, with the soul's desire to embrace God. I felt I was getting at the bottom of all my human desires and felt just with a profound deep desire to love. I felt a love I had never felt ever before. A love that destroys you, an accomplished love as the lover was not present. I was longing for God with all my heart. The pain so intense that It was a soul's pain, a longing, a desperate intent to connect with the lost lover. So much passion, so much deep desire to become one with God.

The vibrations started again and became even stronger. I could hear the murmur, the exquisite secrets spread in my ears. Visions, premonitions and messages came to me. I saw myself rising, I felt myself transforming like emerging from a cocoon. I felt I was finally accepting that I was a spiritual being.

I felt that I was surrendering. I was giving up my body, my perception of self to allow a new force to take over.

A new "me" was emerging, I was spending so many hours in deep meditation. I was disconnecting from reality but this time I did not fight it. I was ready to embrace it.

Most of the time there were no words in my semantics to describe the perceptions. I knew that new areas in my brain where waking up. It was like embracing the Universe. All the calls from childhood, all the attempts to get my attention, my teen years' fears of the energy; all stopped in a breath. A voice said to me: Do nothing!

However, when I was coming back to this reality things were not good. I started dating and it was a disaster. It seemed I was attracting abusers and rude and unkind men. I could not hold a relationship for more than a couple of months as they were nasty pieces of diarrhoea.

I was living on income support and had no idea what to do. I was sure that I did not want to leave Drew by himself. His mama was the only thing he had in the world. I was devoted to that child, I simply adored him.

I wanted something that I could do at home and be able to be with my boy after school hours.

But what to do?

I struggled again and a new crisis began. I was feeling inadequate, unable to be a mystic and single mother at the same time.

My years of yearning to be in a convent was distant. How could I become a spiritual being living in a world of consumerism and mother of a young child with no money, extremely qualified in fields that I did not want to experience ever again.

I had a deep crisis one day where I was feeling so sorry for myself. I felt that Job in the Bible had it easier in comparison to me.

I remember that it was during the day before I had to pick up Drew from his school, that I started having the worse pain ever. I was in the kitchen and I found myself on the floor, crying so much, screaming and shouting to God, Why? Why me? Why all this misery. How much pain can I handle and why? Why God are you doing this to me…? I had given you my life, I surrendered to you. I asked why is everything hopeless, why is there just like a little bit of light and then you take everything away from me…

I hated HIM, I loved HIM… I felt I was dying a thousand times over. The black and white chess tiles, of the cold floor. I could see among the seas of my tears images of my ex-husband's cruelty during my pregnancy when he forced me to spend a night on the kitchen floor. I felt when he pulled me by my long brown hair and dragged me from the bed to the kitchen floor to sleep there as I was taking too much space in the bed (I was six months' pregnant) … I remembered then when he came back and pulled over from underneath of my frightened body the tea towels I put to make it more comfortable and protect my tummy from the cold floor. "YOU sleep there like the animal that you are" with his fist against my eye!… I remembered the dirt under the cooker and saying to myself, "I am so lucky he cannot see it, he will be furious and most probably he will force me to clean it right now"

I felt all the pain from the absurdity of the deliverances that I had been subject to. I felt the pain of my teen years when I could not get anybody to understand me and suffered in silence. I was losing my mind.

I felt the pain of living my life in France and the confusion of my present life. I remembered all my failed romantic adventures and the pain again of being mistreated. The fear that it was me who was attracting this type of loser.

I felt all the pain and suffering at once and the sea of tears was draining out as they could not produce enough to moisten the desert of pain.

Then I thought of Jorge Luis Borges one of my favourite writers and his poem The Game of Chess. Borges was an Argentinian writer, one of the Jewels of Latin-American literature.

He describes the game of chess as the scenario of life itself and the paradox between player and chess pieces that are in an endless battle of hate and destruction. Opposite colours perpetuating a ritual whose amphitheatre is now the whole world.

These players, King and Queen, Bishop or Pawn do not know it is the artful hand of the player that rules their fate subduing their free will. However, the player who manoeuvres his pieces, he is also a pawn, a bishop on another game board of opposites, of black and white squares of dark nights and light days. Then God moves the player and he moves the piece. What God behind that God originates the first scheme perpetuating the pain, the ignorance and the dream?

I screamed at God with all my lungs' pain asking him to show me his move. What should I do oh beloved God?

The next morning in the mail box was a catalogue of local Adult Education schools and there was my sign, Complementary therapies! I got my answer. Finally, I found my move.

I enrolled onto the Holistic Massage diploma in 2006 and I was a natural. It seemed all the years of pre-medicine and microbiology were working as I had an advantage. That was my scientific training. I knew the anatomy and the physiology so I felt I could get a deeper understanding of the healing provided through the massage. It was a revelation to me, how touch could transfer energy and help different areas in the body, mainly pain management, not only physical pain, but stress and emotional pain too.

Finally, after all, I came back to do what I was naturally doing when I was a child. Touching people and animals to make them feel better.

Then I carried on, doing many more courses, Reflexology again, it came very natural to me, even if anatomically it does not have any sense at all in western medicine, but the energy was there. I was resonating with that vibration too. I could feel and tell people where they had problems, even the bodies were telling me things that had happened in the past and that their bodies were still haunted by the memories.

I opened a small practice at home. I bought a massage couch and modified my lounge. I used it as my practice. It was perfect. I could work from home so my boy could have his mum at home. Then I found a programme through the job centre where they were offering free courses to become self-employed. I did the course and I registered my first company as sole trader, Rafa Nissi.

Rafa Nissi came through a meditation. They are Hebrew words, Rafa means God that heals, therefore Saint Raphael Archangel is the angel of healing and Nissi, is the God who supports us, God who is the pillar, the banner that represents us. I thought it was simply perfect. It defined who I was.

Then I did my course of Reiki level I. That was my next step in the spiritual world.

It was life changing. One, if not the most revealing, experience in my whole life.

In Reiki, you get a series of attunements where you are connected to the energy. In Reiki that is the Universal life force. It is a frequency, a vibration that you can channel and transfer at will. This energy is a healing energy that provides life force to whatever part of the body/mind/emotions are needed as it has its own intelligence. Reiki does not use the energy of the "healer" it is just a vehicle to transfer the energy. It came to me so naturally as I have always been a Reiki practitioner.

During the course, there is a meditation where you meet your Reiki Guide(s).

Oh, it was so beautiful. I was moved to my core. That longing of my dark night came fulfilled at that moment in time.

I was so overwhelmed by the experience that I could not contain my tears and even the Reiki teacher felt the intensity of the episode. Hours later I was still in shock and during the lunch hour I could not stop crying out of love and joy.

My master who has always being with me was Jesus Christ. I felt his presence so vivid and I recognised that energy and vibration in the river, in my room while leaving my body, in my teens, in my dark night of the soul.

I had been part of his energy, I finally felt I had found where I belonged.

Then after that more masters came. It was not only Jesus but other wonderful beings who are associated with Buddhism and Hinduism among others.

After that, I never got any more spiritual attacks. I was free of low tormented energies. I stopped seeing them and I could detect their presence and put them away.

I started to explore oriental philosophies and religions. I studied the Gita. I connected so deeply with Paramahansa Yogananda, I understood the spirit of Zen, I felt Buddha's teachings. A whole world opened to me, a deep love grew and a fresh understanding. Osho's readings were more a confirmation in words of what I already knew. I became attracted to Tantra. This divine principle is so full of love and liberation.

There was no more judgment, freedom to feel and no more pain. Of course, I am still experiencing situations of conflict and moments that were disappointing and sad but there was not the attachment. Even I can lose my temper from time to time but there is different vision of the overall picture that becomes universal. I got a divine wisdom. People wonder sometimes how can I know so much. I just tell them I am empty. I am nothingness. I do not carry anything with me, I remember and know nothing (as Socrates was telling me, when I was a child). I just tap into the stream of universal knowledge when you ask a question. If it is for your own healing and benefit the answer you are in need of and able to hear will come through my lips.

I finally was happy being me. Being less and less a me. Whatever is would be and it is okay or not with me.

I carried on studying more and more complementary therapies. I became a Reiki Master and I started teaching spirituality and Reiki.

I became a Spiritual healer as well plus more "down to Earth therapies" such as Sport Massage and Remedial massage. I found Thai Yoga Massage fascinating. It is a wonderful therapy, so powerful and full of energy. Father Doctor Shivaga who was Buddha's physician is the founder of this discipline.

I did courses in Marma therapy with Dr. Ernst Schrott, one of the greatest Ayurveda practitioner in the West. Ernst, who has his practice in Germany, and I became very good friends. He recognised I was taping into energy naturally, he knew that I could hear the marma points that were unbalanced. He has written over 20 books and he is the vice president of the Ayurveda Medicine Association. He told me he has never met anyone like me.

We were exchanging distant healing a lot of times and I could perfectly feel his presence and working in different areas in my body.

Then I did a diploma in Oncology Massage and Reflexology for Cancer patients.

Cancer is something that caught my attention. I had the feeling that I could help Cancer sufferers.

I became a volunteer at the Community Cancer Centre, which was a local small organisation that helps as many people they can with very little resources. I loved working with them as I could see first-hand how much you could do to alleviate the pain and give love and comfort to the patients and their carers and relatives.

I met a few wonderful characters. One of them was my beloved Carol. I loved her so much.

She gave me so much and showed me the way to help others.

Carol was in her early fifties. She was very petite. She had olive skin and beautiful warm, sweet brown eyes. She was a patient with terminal cancer. Doctors gave up on her. They did not even offer her palliative chemotherapy, as they sent her to die like an old dog.

They gave her a few weeks to live but Carol felt differently.

She came to me short of breath and so tired just by doing a few steps. She hugged me and told me: "you have eyes that I can trust".

She took her clothes off and it was very evident where her cancer started. It was breast cancer that have metastasised all over.

Carol had instead of breast a white patch. A rectangular patch like the square of a Teletubby, right in front of her chest. It was a charcoal patch to absorb all the misery of her interstitial fluid, a lymph that cannot stop pouring healing where there is none.

The cancer had consumed her flesh and underneath the patch it was a labyrinth of hell, twisted tumours curving and swirling around in a sinuous movement of death. There was necrotic tissue in dark brown and vivid red colours. Her lymph nodes were swollen like marble beads, hard and pearl like lustrous tones of an exacerbated system fighting until the end.

She was so ashamed of her breasts. She had to keep them covered to avoid infection but there was not a patch that could cover her pain and misery.

She allowed me to have a look as she felt that it was love and compassion and a profound desire to help her. The look in her brown sad eyes staring at me with such humility and in need pierced my memories until now.

We started a very exciting routine. I dropped my other clients and I dedicated myself to helping Carol. She was determined to prove that alternative therapies could help. We started by changing her diet. Nutrition is essential in a healing process. Carol started a vegetarian diet to detoxify the body and make it more alkaline. We used Naturopathic principles which are that health is achievable in an alkaline environment.

We found out the most alkalising food, plus superfoods known to be anticancer. I designed a menu for her and I was cooking for her too. We had dozens of supplements to boost her immune system.

Ernst from Germany got involved and sent Carol Ayurveda medication. He advised us to make hot compresses of Turmeric powder on her chest. I was doing the compresses two to three times a day.

My friend Margaret Karlinski, who is one of the best aromatherapists in the country, made some inhalers and lotions for Carol to help her breathing and to sleep.

I was doing two to three organic coffee enemas in Carol a day. I was massaging her, doing Reflexology, meditation and Reiki every day.

But mainly we talked and talked. She was opening and releasing all the emotions she had keeping for years. She had many issues with one of her daughters mainly as she could not reach her. She loved her family very much but she could not understand her daughter. They fought a lot and Carol felt she was a burden for all of them. Carol had cancer for over 10 years.

She felt guilty as she was a sick mother without much to offer. She was a faint reflection of the shadow of the powerful executive that she used to be. She saw herself as a whisper, a bag of bones with an oxygen tank. She felt her family resented her for being ill for so many years, as she had failed at being a mother and a wife.

Her family loved her and they learnt to live with her cancer. All of them were busy, working or studying. Carol spent the day by herself alone waiting for them to come home tired and hungry to look after her and that was killing her.

We talked and talked and talked until she finally understood that the cancer was hers. She had difficulties in accepting my message.

"Love your life, love your cancer as it is yours. They are your little babies, your lost cells, like young teenagers that went on the wrong path. Look at your chest and see your scars, see them with love and compassion as no one else would do". I said.

"Accept them as part of who you are. We do not fight cancer. We do not create more stress and fear creating an enemy. We can overcome it with love and compassion. It is like turning the other cheek as Jesus was telling in one if his stories".

Cancer is not an enemy, you cannot fight an imaginary war. The first thing is to control your mind, release the fear through acceptance.

By accepting you have cancer it is not giving up. By surrendering to your natural healing process and release fear and stress you are not making the cancer bigger.

Every time when I see the social concept of the war against cancer, to fight the cancer, it makes me so sad, as it should be the opposite. We can deeply relax when there is love, peace, understanding and acceptance. As I see it, already the body is doing as much as it can to create healing mechanisms to destroy cancerous cells. In fact, every day, all of us are doing that. We all have abnormal cells that the body deals with. There are lots of scientific research in naturally occurring spontaneous healing processes that cure cancer. So, we all deal with potential cancerous cells with our immune system. We are not in a war. We are in a synchronised harmonious process working within our bodies. Sometimes, it does not work as well as it should and then we need to work alongside the body in a team and not against it.

Stress and fear and being in a state of fight makes things worse.

We need to create empowerment through love and compassion after all the cancer cells are yours, they belong to you, to your body.

We work better in teams so what better team than the one with your own self?

It took a while to Carol to feel love for her chest, to allow fresh air and sunlight to caress it. We used to go to her back garden where she sunbathed without the patch.

We observed it, we got familiar with it and we accepted it. It was not repugnant anymore. We were allowing the imagination to play with her chest like a blank canvas giving names and shapes to the different areas of the labyrinth through love and compassion that needed to be felt and not just kept as an intellectual concept.

I taught Carol to feel with her mind and to think with her heart.

A few weeks later Carol made improvements. She started gaining weight and got more animated. The production of fluids and the death tissue on her chest were reducing, it was getting dry and had a better colour. Carol was breathing without the need to use her Oxygen tank. There was no pain. She had a better appetite and was sleeping better.

Her dream was opening a centre for alternative therapies, a hospice with all the treatments to make people better. She became my best advocate. She was more motivated to go out and even started wearing make-up. She made peace with her cancer and celebrated life. This time it did not matter for how long as she was not in a race anymore.

Some of her relatives came from abroad to visit her and she was less in need of my vigilant services. I explained to all of them to carry on with the compresses and with the enemas at least once a day, but my efforts fell on deaf ears. It seemed suddenly they knew better.

Also, it was time for me to go back to my practice as money was very low as Carol could not afford my services and I had my own obligations to cover too.

Carol was enjoying that summer, she was happy and that was the only thing that was important.

But no one was doing the compresses or the enemas and they found the supplements were far too many and too expensive…

She called me a couple of months later, as she was deteriorating again. I went to see her but I felt her end was approaching. The bluesish white hard marble pearls that went down once came bigger and now they were in her head too.

She started doing the compresses herself but she was getting very tired and not able to do all the things we did together. And that it is the problem with alternative treatments, it requires constant sacrifice and very hard work.

Chemotherapy and Radiotherapy are very passive therapies. They kill you but you are a passive recipient where doctors and nurses take the power from you and dictate what you must do or not to do.

You deal with the effects of the poison with side effects and you become a victim. So again, a passive disposition, they are the side effects that stoically we need to endure.

You are a casualty of the fight against cancer. The WAR on Cancer is destroying you and you must fight, fight, fight! As if dealing with the poison alone of the treatment was not hard enough!

But in this life, everyone has the right to choose the treatment they trust best. You need to feel reassured and able to trust. The ideal is that you put the trust in yourself! After all, it is your life, it is your cancer and it is your death too. I have worked with a lot of cancer patients and brain tumour patients. My work is more an integrative therapy than alternative but I have seen how much the therapies help not only the patients but their relatives and carers too.

Carol called me for the last time a few weeks later disorientated and feeling lost with palpitations. She had called an ambulance and wanted to hear my voice while she was waiting for the ambulance, she told me she was far too tired to carry on. I told her it was okay.

She was entitled to give up and to rest. We both knew it was a good-bye call. Despite that she was so afraid and wanted to get a second glance at hope. I found myself bringing it to her through kind words "it is okay, whatever happens you are going to be more than okay. Go to the hospital my sweet friend you will see all will be fine". There was no need to say anything differently than that.

She had made her peace with death a while ago in our afternoon long conversations. She made peace with her daughter's attitude too. She would not change her anger and she would not feel guilty anymore.

A few days later she died at the hospital of a cardiac arrest.

I love Carol and I am so grateful to her. I learnt so much with her and my heart became humble and grateful for her generosity and friendship. She allowed me to be part of her last months of her life.

Carol lived extra 5 months of what all the doctors predicted with a modest improvement in her quality of life for some but for her she felt alive again.

Working with Carol was a privileged experience. One of the most fulfilling and humbling ones. There was so much love, truth, soul. The unravelling of all that it is fake and unneeded. The core soul loving life and making sense and acceptance of death. Her kind generosity that chose and trusted me to be a witness of her beautiful spirit. Only gratitude and love I have for that beautiful woman who gave me beautiful lesson of life. Understanding life through the process of death is a unique experience that she so generously offered to me.

When I was working at the Cancer Centre I met Doug. Doug was a tiny old Jamaican personage. He was in remission from Prostate cancer.

He was so funny and proud of his physical appearance. He spontaneously was showing you he could touch his toes by bending over with straight knees.

He had the most contagious laugh and was so witty and funny. He became my most regular client, coming for years to my little practice at home. We created a routine. He arrived early for his appointment and cooked for us lunch. A wonderful shrimp's soup. A little Caribbean treasure full of love and joy, made with exotic vegetables and a hint of kindness and heat.

Then after our lunch we played Dominos. He was a regional champion on his good days and it was so rewarding seeing a little glance of wickedness and cheekiness every time he saw I was trying so hard to win with no success.

It is so wonderful when your clients become your friends and he was a real loyal friend. For years, I treated him, then I felt things were going down the drain. He was getting older but to me it was something more than that. He was feeling as he used to say to me "rough".

I needed to do something; I spoke to his daughter and I suggested that he needed to be checked to see if the cancer was back. I did not want to scare her and neither was I doing a diagnosis but I felt the cancer was back for a while and I had to say something.

A few days later she called me and said she went to the GP and did some blood tests but he was just having a little bit of anaemia. A week later she called me and said to me her father had a stroke and it came out he had a terminal Cancer that affected his brain too. He died shortly after that.

It was hard to lose Doug, I am still picturing him touching his toes and showing me how fit he was. He was not the only personal loss that I had in 2015. My best friend and my business partner, Rod also started with a funny little cough. I started feeling the same feeling that I felt before. He got kidney cancer that had spread to his liver and lungs.

Before the doctor made the diagnosis, I knew it and I told my mother in tears that Rod will not make it. I said to her in May 2015, I feel he has cancer and would not pass November. My beloved best friend died in the early days of November as I predicted. I knew no matter whatever he did he would not make it. During Reiki treatments, it was so evident that death was there and nothing could be done. I never said anything to him and it was so painful to feel his life was going away. My beloved Rod was so generous that he allowed me, just a few hours before his death when he was in the coma, to be there next to him. I saw his soul and saw a light and he was holding back as he did not want to leave me alone, I heard his voice apologising to me as he let me down, he knew that he was my rock that I needed his help so much, I said good bye to my best friend, that it was okay for him to go.

I sent him Reiki at that moment to help him to detach himself of his duty and I felt so much love. I saw beings of light around him. He died a few minutes after I left the hospital.

While I was studying my Oncology Massage course I did a lot of research about the different aspects that can affect your health and how to heal yourself. One of these studies was based on neuroplasticity and neuropsychology. How your beliefs can affect your physical body and your health.

I studied other principles that the body talks to you and that there are emotional/mental connections to the illnesses we manifest.

An example of that is in the lovely book of Louise Hay. She explains the root cause of different conditions and how by using different affirmations we can condition our mind to change our beliefs and by modifying our own beliefs we can heal ourselves. She based her affirmation on stating that you must love yourself first then you can add what you want to achieve. Wonderfully simple and efficient.

Also, the effects of meditation and the changes that this mental discipline has on the physiology of the body and brain triggering changes in behaviour and beliefs. We evolve through our own perceptions and our brain adapts accordingly. Our health is based on our beliefs as chemical reactions are triggered through our neurotransmitters that are orchestrated in our brain. Stress factors can be modulated in our own psychodrama as their perception is a creation of the mind.

I also checked some studies in naturopathy and alkalising diets to detoxify the body. The principle is that the more acidic the body is the more toxic it is and that cancer develops easier in acidic environments and makes the body acidic. I based the diet that I made to Carol and other Cancer patients on naturopathy.

I also did research on how other cultures worked out their own healing systems. I found Ayurveda, the Indian healing system that works with harmony and balance. A mix of energy work and the use of nature.

An area in Ayurveda caught my attention as it is based on energy work; the chakras, the nadis, marmas to name a few. Ayurveda refers to the relationship between our bodies and the connection with the universe. We are part of a whole universe, a vital energy called Prana that is a life force. In Reiki, also we work with energy, Ki or Chi that is this flow of life.

In this relationship, Ayurveda works with geometrical features called Yantras, a universal language with its own vibrations that connects with our energy centres. Also, they work with Rudrakshas, a holy seed that the Hindu tradition says are the tears of Lord Shiva. When Lord Shiva heard about the human suffering he wept and his tears fell on the ground and this tree was born to help to overcome the sorrows.

The Rudrakshas have different sizes, like satsumas with different segments and they go from 1 segment (Mukhis) to 21 Mukhis.

Each one of these segments resonates with the energy of the chakras that are energy centres, vortexes that rotate like dynamos generating life force bringing harmony, health, happiness, awareness and prosperity to one's life.

Each chakra brings a main life lesson and represents different physical, mental and emotional aspects in our own life but also relationships and how we interact with others.

There are seven major chakras in the body; root, sacral, solar plexus, heart, throat, third eye and crown.

Ayurveda also works with Ratna or gems using the same principle, as each stone has different properties and chemical composition which has a different energy that interacts with ours and with the Universe. All the gems, Rudrakshas, Yantras have an interaction with astrology and Hinduism.

A fabulous combination of quantum physics, geometry, chemistry, mythology and psychology in a cultural tradition that dates thousands of years ago, at the grasp of our hands.

In December 2013, after a deep meditation I searched on the internet for Yantras. I saw in my mind during the meditation the geometrical shape, a pyramid with different layers and sequences that has a vibration.

I found a website, Rudraksha Ratna in India that has the most beautiful pieces. Tri dimensional ones carved in different stones.

As soon I saw them I could feel their vibration a different tone and the whole website was so strong, a wonderful force emanating from it. I could not stop reading about each one as the whole information was simply fascinating.

It felt pure, holy and honest. It was the genuine desire to honour and serve the energies. The company belongs to Neeta Singhal, an amazing lady with a wonderful presence and knowledge.

I bought three Yantras, one in Rose quartz, a second one in Aventurine and a third one in Citrine.

As soon as I got them I felt a shift, like my own energy was getting a boost, the frequency of the vibration has changed.

By then my hope was to upgrade my little practice and relocate out of my house. But of course, I did not have the money to do so. Despite my efforts, I had only a few clients, around 5 a week when lucky and living on tax credits and benefits.

Then soon after I got the Yantras things started to change, it was a possibility for things to change.

A couple of clients of mine offered help and lent me money, Rod also agreed to be my partner and helped me so much. Other friends gave me their support and money. Different schemes and possible partnerships became a reality in a matter of days.

Then, it was a surreal atmosphere, nothing in concrete but buzzing and witnessing synchronicity in each step like steering a ship in turbulent waters, one move at the time and taking decisions so fast without even knowing how I would pay for it. A client suggested Pinner in Harrow. It was just half of an hour drive from home and a charming little place like a chocolate box picture frozen in time and afar from busy maniac London life. I loved the place straight away and there were by then so many empty premises on the high street to choose from.

We visited a few but nothing looked right for what I had in mind, suddenly it was there, waiting for me, I felt the energy of the place was calling me. It was not very big and it had been empty for a few years but I knew it was the place to start the healing process.

Again, during meditation, the name of Spatium came to my mind. And in March 2014 Spatium was created and officially registered in the Company House. I was the director of my own limited company and all the years of studies in such variety of subjects, business, arts, sciences finally came in handy.

Spatium means space in Latin. A space in physical terms but also in time; a tempo, a period, a frequency of time and it is an anatomical term to describe inner space among the tissues.

Finally, my dream to provide a space to heal was taking shape. My objective was to provide different disciplines under the same roof of Alternative and Complementary Medicine, therefore the name Spatium ACM.

It was a new start, a small place with a big challenge, but it was my vocation, the force that drives me every day, to be able to help people to feel better.

I bought the franchise of the Rudraksha Ratna, I got the exclusivity for the UK of their amazing products and I got trained by Neeta, helping people to balance their chakras. I found another dimension and a deeper connection into the energy field of the person and it had increased my psychic levels to help them.

I realised that I can use my sensitivity to energies and provide insight for healing purposes.

I designed the place and logos, marketing, prices. I was applying all the years of eclectic knowledge. I had several issues and problems and fights with people who are no longer part of the business. I also, lost my beloved Rod to death.

I struggled with money issues as the place despite being so good and feeling charged with the most amazing healing energy has not made a profit. I had to finance the place with even more personal loans, overdrafts, credit cards, and not able to pay myself a salary every month but there is compelling force that drives me to carry on.

I had so many testimonials from people who came for help and how this love and compassion has made a difference in their lives, that it has encouraged me to carry on.

One of the most touching experiences was Mina. Mina has a recurrent lung cancer and was in a bad place when she contacted me.

I am sharing with you a letter she wrote to me:

"Dear Adriana

I am writing to tell you how grateful I am to you, for everything you have done, everything you are doing and everything I am still yet to experience and benefit from.

Words cannot express the experience I have with you, the journey you are taking me on is so wonderful and amazing.

As you are aware, I was diagnosed with lung cancer – stage 4 – in November 2014. The Oncologist has given me two years to live. With such devastating news, you can imagine how I felt emotionally. I started treatment in December 2014 and by March 2015, it had cleared up. Unfortunately, when I went back for my 3 month CT scan at the end of July, it was discovered that my cancer had returned in my Lymph nodes in the right lung.

On the 8th November 2015, a day I will never forget, as I was at my lowest point of giving up and I was in such an emotional state as that whole week was full of negativity for me and someone close to me had just passed away of cancer. I just didn't know who to turn to or talk to about how I was feeling. Then suddenly, your name came into my head and I knew I had to call you.

After speaking to you on the phone, Adriana, I HAD A VISION OF HOPE.

On Thursday 12th November 2015, I got my first appointment with you. WOW... How amazing and wonderful I felt. YOU were so connected with my MIND...... BODY........ &..... SOUL. I left your clinic feeling as if the weight has been lifted off my shoulders. I felt as I could stand up straight and walk into the path of HOPE AND STRENGH AND POSITIVITY.

I went home and thought about everything you did and said to me. Encouraging me, supporting me and most of all and very importantly... UNDERSTANDING ME.

I have now had 4 sessions with you and I feel so POSITIVE and HAPPY knowing that I will beat this cancer. Like you said to me…… EMBRACE the cancer… and only then, can you CONTROL the cancer.

I have adopted this attitude and I feel like a completely new person. I feel as if I have been RE-BORN again. I have been given a new lease of LIFE. I am taking this opportunity and EMBRACING it with both hands.

I believe that GOD sent you to me so TOGETHER WE ARE GOING ON MY JOURNEY OF RECOVERY.

THANK YOU SO MUCH 'ADRIANA' FROM THE BOTTOM OF MY HEART.

GOD BLESS YOU"

Mina Andrews

Like Mina, I have several testimonials that are not only related to Cancer. I have my Reiki students who all of them have experienced different changes in their lives. I love teaching and provide guidance and wisdom to those who are in need.

One of my students is David. He became one of my protégées as I see in him so much potential. He has given so much and finally he is shifting from a life of suffering to self-awareness and peace.

David had issues with drugs and alcohol. He was in his late twenties but behaved much younger than his physical age. His mind was a teenager, a mini Peter Pan refusing to contemplate an image of one growing up.

He was in pain and in distress as the contradiction of his nature antagonised with his lifestyle. David was a spiritual being, with great potential, a beautiful caring soul with a difficult upbringing.

He was dyslexic which did not help in his intellectual capacities. Also, his mother was an alcoholic.

His father worked abroad and was providing financial support, but David was feeling neglected and abandoned.

His mother's drinking was escalating so much and getting out of control. She wanted a drinking buddy and was pleased to see her son drinking with her. He turned to drugs and alcohol when he was a teenager and when I met him he was in rehab.

David was passing by and was attracted by Spatium's energy. As soon he entered he felt so good, happy and safe. He was attracted to chakras and just recently he was learning about them.

He came to show me a tattoo he had with the chakras! We connected straight away and I felt his pain and mental confusion.

He came for one of my chakra readings and bought the Rudrakshas that I recommended for him to wear. He felt an instant release and a force supporting him from day one.

David decided to become one of my Reiki students and I attuned him into this energy. His life started to change in front of his own eyes. His addiction was more under control to the point that he felt no desire, nor need to take drugs. His alcohol intake also gradually reduced. He started seeing life differently, from a different perspective. He was feeling unconditional love not only for others but most important for himself.

David gained day by day more self-esteem and his peers were noticing it. He had issues with relationships with young ladies as most of them did not see him as a potential candidate to be in love with, so my poor sweet David was pouring his love like a desperate abandoned puppy dog. He was being so needy that his feelings were crushed and his confidence again down the drain.

I was so happy to see David looking into his inner self and getting stronger from the core. His mother was deteriorating and they had a lot of conflicts as he loved her and she was self-destroying. He was assuming her role of being the protector, the guide in the family.

There were so many emotions in place. In these situations, it is easy to deny or to confuse them. There was anger, love, resentfulness, frustration, temptation. There were moments of joy, fun and darkness and depression. Loneliness and feeling the whole world was on his shoulders, as he was the carer of someone who did not want to be cared for. Moments of lies and denial, turning away as reality was not good.

He was working in a restaurant as a waiter which he really hated and was not particularly good at. He had a degree in Psychology, looking after an alcoholic and being himself an addict too.

Then David realised he was different. He was a very sensitive being to energies. He was a psychic, a naturally gifted healer. He had so many manifestations that scared him and he used to come to visit me asking for guidance and reassurance. David was flourishing in front of my eyes. He was teaching his friends about spirituality, about meditation, about Reiki. He started to treat them with Reiki and some of them came to me for Chakra readings, talks and Reiki too.

His relationship with his mother improved. Unfortunately, in 2016 she died of liver failure caused by her alcoholism. Her passing was a very special moment. I met her a few weeks before she went to the hospital. She came to see me and we had a conversation. I treated her and I told her if she did not stop drinking right there she would die soon. It was her choice to face the pain and the shame of her addiction and face forgiveness, and stop the sorrow and self-pity or die.

Sometimes, pain and dislike of one's self is the easiest choice to make as to forgive oneself is the most difficult part when we know that we have caused so much pain and damage to others.

Guilt is an emotion that destroys you. The guilt of a mother is even higher as the role we play means to be sacred. We bring beings into the world, giving life and sometimes we measure our role accordingly against the success and happiness of our children.

There is no sharper blade than the feeling of letting down our own children. The shame, the pain of causing them harm or guiding them into the wrong direction. To feel responsible for their unhappiness and failures.

How many darts of pain we throw to our own heart, darts of blame and excuses for every action taken and those we did not take. Then a second wave of attacks, in our inner dialogues of the possible "If" I did so, or If I do so and so…. As "If" would be a real hypothesis, a parallel reality that I am to blame for not happening. As "IF" was the powerful tool to instigate more pain. IF is a conditional, it needs something else to be a reality, so by definition, it does not exist alone.

We all fall into these mental dramatic plays, sooner or later we are playing all the roles, and the mind really enjoys their "telenovelas", their soap operas to entertain us. The more dramatic the more fun we have.

It is up to us to tune up or down the drama of our own experiences. The mind has been trained by evolution to think of the worst-case scenario and tends to have the negative side at hand to prepare the mechanism to defend herself. It is part of your genetic imprint from thousands of years of evolution. An animal that is a prey and equally a predator must be vigilant and expect the unexpected to survive. The moments of joy and relaxation under the sun are limited and someone in the tribe is on the lookout. Fight and flight reaction is intrinsic to our endocrine system and it plays a role in your mind. The dinosaurs have left us but our fears have stayed.

Our predators and our prey are emotional. Emotions are energies that we trigger and store in our bodies. It is our choice to determine how we are going to deal with them.

We can play the roles of predator and prey all our lives and both roles at the same time to our own self and to others. That inner dialogue, that corrodes your mind, the darts of pain that recreate so many negative scenarios of your own self preying on others and self-destroying your own soul.

Our brains have the ability to change patterns of behaviours and beliefs by the transformation of the inner mind's dialogue. Our soul, that intrinsic definition of the self, connects through our mind, a conductor of vibrational communication, the energy that transforms the physical structure that it is our brain, triggering by biochemical reactions synapsis sending messages to our whole self, the physical body, mind, emotions, in sum to what we perceive and believe define us consciously and unconsciously.

There is this beautiful book for those who may be interested in the more scientific semantical explanation on how we work. It is Buddha's Brain, the practical neuroscience of happiness, love and wisdom by the doctors Rick Hanson and Richard Mendius.

David's mother had a choice. She decided to die as her pain of being an alcoholic and self-judgment of being a bad mother was stronger than the positive messages of forgiveness and love for one's self.

Her mind denied the possibility of changing her synapsis. It was her choice, and it was okay. We all have choices and we all assume their consequences. The wonderful thing that in her heart of loving mother she took a few weeks to die. Time was her gift for her husband to come back home and play the role of father and husband. Time that allowed the children to feel a deep love and forgiveness for their dying mother. Love and compassion and understanding came across and they had time to share and to talk, to love, to hate and to cry. They started the mourning process with her alive that helped them to learn about their own feelings and to accept them.

It was when she felt that there was no more she could do to make peace with her loved ones that she passed away.

David learnt that he was not a mini Peter Pan anymore. He realised his father loved him and his mother was special to him in her own way and the resentfulness and pain were less. Of course, waves of sadness come time to time as the mourning process is still going on.

He is now working with an organisation that cares for mentally disabled individuals and is in a stable relationship. He is a Reiki practitioner and a very knowledgeable meditator. His perception of his life changed and he is in a better place to handle life in all its splendour. He is still smoking and going to his rock concerts and perhaps partying here and there but the pain is gone, the lack of love for himself is gone too.

I have helped thousands of people, some of them just coming to see me for physical ailments, tired muscles, stress and fatigue. Others with emotional, spiritual or mental pains. The level of needs does not matter, as I am always there for people.

Most of my clients tell me that I have miraculous healing hands. They are amazed that I seem to know what is wrong with them before they open their mouth. That my hands know where their pain is. Some of them even get scared when I tell them episodes of their life that they need to sort out. I just tell them what their body is telling me. We all have the faculty to listen to our own bodies, we just need to have a quieter mind to do so.

Only a couple of times I have confronted very negative spirits, casting them out from their host. I have gone to houses to clear the energies to reassure their residents. I am also a Spiritual Healer although it is not my favourite therapy. I prefer to work with other types of energies.

I am so lucky to count on an astounding team of fantastic professionals working alongside me with the same ethos and goodness of heart.

Yvonne Sarratt is an amazing sensitive lady who has dedicated her life helping children and young adults and their mental health. She is very energy orientated and can understand, feel and communicate with young beings. Her rate of success is very high. She also works with adults and supervises other psychotherapists.

We have great plans and projects to develop to help children. We want to create a holistic programme integrating psychotherapy with complementary therapies and other activities such as arts, gardening, sports, interaction with other generations and providing a social value to our teenagers. We want to change the perception of isolation and bring unconditional love to these youngsters who are labelled under the Tier 2 category! These children are sensitive ones that for one reason or another they are depressed, withdrawn, unable to integrate, self-harming amongst other manifestations. These children are not ill or bad enough to be part of the health system designed for mental health CAMHS (Child and Adolescent Mental Health Services), but their pain is real and they find themselves with no help.

Our dream is to be able to create a space for these children and a training academy for psychotherapists and counsellors to understand and work with young individuals in a holistic open minded way.

Margreet Souren is unique. She is also a complementary therapist like me. We studied together and trained for several years in different disciplines. She is Dutch and is so tall that I feel like a little mouse next to her. She is also a Reiki practitioner and has a lovely and caring cheerful disposition to life.

Quyen Tran is our Chinese Medicine practitioner and Acupuncturist and Reiki practitioner too. She is simply magnificent in what she does. She is extremely competent with vast knowledge and so passionate about her trade. Quyen is from Vietnam and has a witty, fresh and direct sense of humour. Buddhist and soft yet powerful in her healing.

Lisa Carroll is a Master Cognitive Hypnotherapist, Havening, Psy-Tap, TFT, NLP, Reiki practitioner and so many more qualifications. She is of Irish descent and vegan. Again, her integrity and sense of care for others is so admirable.

Orazio Giuffrida is our doctor in Neuropsychology and Memory clinic practitioner. Orazio works in several NHS hospitals. He is Italian, from Sicily, with a lovely pleasant accent.

We also count on the collaboration of Maria West who is our Mindfulness practitioner. She mainly works with children. She has devoted years in understanding the young mind. Maria has such a kind, giving generous heart, spiritual and charitable, helping as many people she can reach.

We also have Anna Winek from Poland, our Naturopathic Nutritionist. She is also another person who is so special, loving and caring committed to her profession.

Varsha Vanaji is a clinical Herbalist with a scientific acumen in Eastern, Chinese and Western herbs. Also, we have Natalia Sayers who is our Kundalini Yoga teacher. Natalia is from Russia. She also excels in her field. She offers sound therapy after her yoga classes, offering a mix of vibrational sounds from Gongs, Tibetan bowls, forks among others.

Then, we have Sara Fisher, our Jewish English Rose, who is our Art teacher and Reiki practitioner. Sara is of an imaginable candour, soft and kind.

I also count on the lovely, caring Aiman Merali, who is an adult counsellor and our Muslim member of the team.

I love working with such a variety of nationalities and cultures. I learn from each one of them. I feel enriched and grateful working with all of them.

One afternoon in October 2016, I was at Spatium working at the reception. Margreet and as usual we were laughing and having a great relaxing time.

The telephone rang and I answered in my accustomed manner.

"Hello, Spatium Clinic, Adriana speaking, how may I help you?"

Then tick... tock... tick......... tock. A voice that took me by surprise. It was a mix of an old fashioned western movie sound, the histrionic voice of John Wayne blended with Humphrey Bogart's Yankee accent. A nasal sound, a deep pitch that drops down at the end of each word.

The last time that I heard that voice on the phone was in 2012 when he called me to tell me his mother, my beloved mother in law, had died.

Margreet saw my face, and the atmosphere changed. I moved my lips to let her know that It was my ex-husband.

Yes, 4 years had passed since his infamous sordid life touched me.

After my divorce, my ex-husband lost his job in the City and moved to Russia to live with his girlfriend in her native Saint Petersburg. I was not in contact with him but always people kept me informed of his moves.

Barbara, his mother, was still in contact. We were good friends and she adored her grandson. I always made sure that my Drew had his grandparents, I divorced her son but not them.

Barbara was married to Todd, her second husband who was such a loving, caring, sweet man. Todd was of a humbler origin than Barbara and a widower who raised 5 children. Barbara divorced my ex-husband's father many years ago, who was another banker and another alcoholic.

They adored Drew and I visited them a few times in Palm Beach and in Long Island.

Barbara never made a financial contribution to us, she never helped us with any of our expenses not even when I was visiting her.

On several occasions, she told me she would make sure Drew would have his education fees paid, and she would provide for that. She would make sure her grandson would have a good start in life. Unfortunately, her words were just words, she never provided for him either death or alive, as she did not mention it in her will.

She was always afraid of not having enough, that money would run out and she would not be able to finance her lifestyle. I never asked for a penny as I knew the answer would be "I cannot afford it".

Then I heard that my ex-husband had moved to Cyprus, this time as a married man, with his Russian lady. We never heard from him, not even an email or a Christmas card. He lived there only for a few years as it seemed he had lost his job.

He then moved to Holland and was working in another bank until again he lost his job. After that, he went back to his mum's, jobless and with his wife.

He then moved to Florida, living under his mum's protection as he had always done. She had bailed him out all his life!

How sad to reach nearly 60 years old and going back to mama. Nevertheless, there were worse place to go, who could not enjoy being in a beautiful house with gardens, an individual pool and at 50 yards from the beach, in Gulf Stream, in Palm Beach!

Barbara had a very bad year. Her husband was diagnosed with Dementia, her best friend and brother in law died. Her youngest sister also died of cancer in a matter of weeks and her son, of whom she was afraid, was living with her. He and his wife were penniless but drinking, smoking and taking drugs as usual.

Barbara was getting ill and she was diagnosed with Kidney Cancer stage 4. It was terminal and spreading very fast to liver and lungs.

I offered my humble services to go and look after her but my offer was received with all possible insults that I had forgotten existed.

The situation was getting worse. He was attacking his own moribund mother, battering her, demanding her to die as soon as possible as he could not wait to get his hands on his mansion.

His wife was wearing Barbara's jewellery without her permission and they were both making the old lady's life miserable.

It got so bad that one day Barbara ran away from home and collapsed in the middle of the road. The paramedics alerted the police as Barbara told them her son had attacked her and that he wanted her dead.

Finally, the police in Palm Beach arrested him for battering the elderly… his own mother!

It was the 24th December and the man spent the night in jail and was bailed for Christmas. There was an injunction forbidding him to be less than 100 yards from his mother.

Barbara rented a small flat for him and his wife to move to, but they refused as it was not good enough for them. So, she decided to leave the house and move to a hospice.

She was dying and in the last days of her life, she changed her will and left her house in Florida to her husband and his children with all its contents, shares and cash too.

To her son, she left a house in Maine and cash of a total of over half of million dollars.

My ex-husband was so angry that he refused to go to her funeral. He was legally evicted months later by his step siblings as it was his mansion no more!

Now, he was on the phone talking to me. I came back to my present and then I witnessed my own transformation. It was an initial moment of surprise and confusion as my brain did not know how to react but then there was peace.

There was not fear just my inner peace radiating unconditional love and compassion.

He was flattering me, on how proud he was of my achievements. He told me that he had been living in London for the past 6 months as he was working on a contract but he could not renew it and he was out of work.

He told me he was temporarily living at one of his friends' house but he needed to move and that he had financial difficulties and could not afford to pay for any accommodation. He wondered if I could lodge him for a few days as he was waiting for his Russian visa so that he could join his wife in Russia where she was living.

I felt sorry for him. I felt compelled to help him. I told him that I needed to discuss the situation with Drew as he was the one who would take the decision to have him at home or not.

Drew was wonderful, I explained the situation and he just said, "Mum, I feel sorry for that man, it is sad he is homeless but please mum, I do not want to be mean but I cannot stand the idea to be under the same roof with that man. I hope you understand, I wish him well and I hope his situation improves but not here mum please" I promised my son that his welfare was my sole priority and I was there to protect him and I would never do anything to cause him harm.

I tried with friends to see if someone would have him and I contacted one of my closest friends who lives up north to see if he could lodge him but my ex-husband refused the idea as it was too far from London. After that I did not hear from him anymore.

I felt that I have finally closed a chapter that lasted 18 years, from the moment I married him in October 1998 to his phone call asking me for help. Money did not talk anymore…

For many years, I asked God to make justice, to grant me the solace and see fairness. I got my moment and it was at the perfect time of my life as I was full of love, peace and compassion that I shared with the man who had hurt me so much. I finally had forgiven and had given away my pain. I indeed understood that to forgive is FOR - GIVE and not FOR - KEEP.

I realised that I have for-given and that I was free!

I am still living in my little housing association house with my beloved children. My beloved Drew and my canine son who is my loyal companion, my adored Topper, a Yellow Labrador who is eleven years old.

PART 2

Concepts and comments

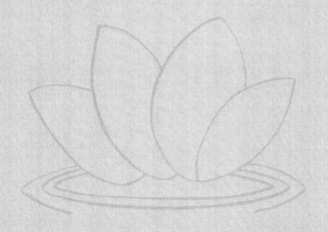

At the beginning of this book I asked you WHY?

And the answer to that one is simply because you deserve it.

Independently of what you are, do, believe, genre, colour, size, age, etc., you just deserve it. You need to do nothing to deserve it.

It is simply not UP TO YOU! Being in harmony, in peace, in unconditional love, in freedom do not have anything to do with what you may or may not do!

You are alive, and life is the answer. It is quintessential for life to strive and prolong its existence. Life is part of the conscious manifestation of the Universe and you are part of it.

Now, to become a manifestation of that energy a wonderful thing happened, two cells have collided and fused to become one, like an atomic bomb!

The level of energy for this to happen is extraordinary. Starting from the beginning, when a female and a male mate they reach a high level of arousal that embraces cosmic energy.

In Tantra, we believe that sexual energy is a creative force, a powerful force that manifests from the lower chakras, from the root that keeps us on the ground travelling through the body in ecstasy and reaches the Universe. It is higher and stronger than us and it connects us to the creator of all. We become connected and we sublimate that force that creates and we procreate. It is a sacred powerful energy, that allows us to create, not only little mini us, but any act of creativity.

This energy is sublime and put us at God's level. When we entwine our sexual energy to become one with a force of creation we are at peace, in harmony, in freedom; only love and compassion can emanate from this holy union. We fuse with love, with God, with the Universe, then we remember we are all ONE.

When you are in your orgasm, you are not anymore with a sexual partner, you forget his eyes, his name, his body, you transcend and become one with the Universe. You are in communion with God in pleasure and in an ecstasy so intense that stops you, in time and space, cutting your breath.

It feels like being a witness of the Big Bang, a creative force that fuses you and completes you. Just realise what is involved to create a new life!

Biologically, the transformation is incredible. An orchestra in unison, in perfect synchronicity, perfect timing and tempo. What are the odds, that an egg that has been formed while your mother was in the uterus of her own mother, matured and travelled through the fallopian tubes then descended to the uterus where it is attacked by millions of missiles!

These little missiles, like tadpoles are so vibrant and full of movement. For a moment think of your father's sperm, the efforts and input of energy that the body has done to produce them. The biochemistry, the right number of nutrients, vitamins and minerals. Semen is only one percent DNA material; the rest is composed of over 200 separate proteins, as well as vitamins and minerals including vitamin C, calcium, chlorine, citric acid, fructose, lactic acid, magnesium, nitrogen, phosphorus, potassium, sodium, vitamin B12, and zinc.

And that is not all. Imagine the process of erection, the hydraulics and physics involved in such mechanism that can be triggered at will through neurochemical messengers from your brain to create the power, that is not more than the acceleration of the energy in movement, to ejaculate. The speed and the competition, a literal race for life.

Each one of these little missiles has 50% of your genetical information, the most efficient mobile microchip, a technology that not Microsoft or Apple can even imagine, the whole history of life in a mini tadpole that is capable of fusing its programme to another in perfect harmony.

Then, the special coating that egg has, that just allows the strongest and the fittest to penetrate it. Then it seals itself in to become a fortress and then the two cells who had transformed themselves through the process of Meiosis where they had only half of their chromosomes paired up to become one. They had the whole history of life in their genome.

Then, the process starts, they copy and divide themselves through Mitosis at an exponential rate. From one to two, to 4, to trillions of cells. They start to differentiate and create different functions accordingly to the position where they are, internal ones grow different organs of your body, the external ones provide limbs and skin and so on. This is perhaps when the term location, location, location was born as it will determine the status of the cells.

In this process of gestation anything can go wrong. Cells cannot differentiate properly. Mitosis can create wrong copies and generate mutations or instead of dividing into two daughter cells can create a multiple of them creating tumours, apoptosis (term for suicidal cells that trigger a mechanism for self-destruction when something did not go as it should be). External factors can trigger changes, life is precarious and powerful at the same time. Everything is possible like in quantum physics.

The foetus evolves and grows, it develops sexual organs and becomes biologically a he or a she, in this case it becomes YOU.

Then, after the period of gestation you are born, a new experience, a new reality and a different environment. You grow and become a child, a teenager and adult, an elderly and you die. A natural process that can be affected at any time.

Can you see all the energy that it is involved in producing a YOU? And for a second expand your thinking and see that the interaction of this embryo is not only to its mum but to the Universe itself.

The composition, the raw materials are chemical elements with an energy charge, a star dust, common to everything in the planet, in the galaxies in the Universe as we understand it.

The carbons, the hydrogens, the oxygens, the nitrogen and so on are the same in a rock, in our oceans, in our streams, in our trees, in our grass, in our soils, in the bacteria, virus, whales and elephants and in the air we breathe.

How beautiful it is to realise we are all one and we are connected as the trees are connected through the soil, through their root systems we are connected to the whole universe, to every living and not living element in our beautiful planet that oozes life in all its splendour.

I invite you to contemplate nature and feel that vibration of love that connects you, please look at the trees, woods, rivers and feel that sense of love, connection and joy. Feel proud to belong after all we are all related to beauty. Feel the desire to protect them as your own children, admire their life force and remember they are transiting through the same process of your own creation.

Each living organism has a process of procreation. A universal explosion of vibrational energy that we understand as life. There is not a colour, a genre, a religion, a good and bad, rich and poor, we all have a biological process that carries all our lives. Honour your life and others and you will be a step ahead of suffering.

Right now, as you are reading this book, perhaps do not realise that your cells are duplicating and dying constantly. Your blood cells, your skin, the lining of your guts, your bones, your liver, your muscles are repairing themselves, your body is digesting and metabolising and your brain, your brain is creating paths of communication, channels that convey messages from your soul, mind to brain and body.

We can mould our brain and therefore alter our biological processes. Positive affirmation and loving and caring thoughts trigger different hormones (chemical communicators) that affect your responses. The positive thoughts generate healing, negative thoughts generate toxins. We need to train the mind with the view to alter the brain paths and be able to do things differently. It becomes a mental exercise that has been performed over thousands of years by Eastern cultures based on observation, contemplation of nature and meditation.

The brain responds to the semantics that the mind is constantly sharing with it. Soul is manifesting through the mind, how much we perceive of it depends on the level of control over the mind.

I found the Gita fascinating (Bhagavad Gita, a 700-verse Hindu scripture in Sanskrit that is part of the Hindu epic Mahabharata (chapters 25 - 42 of the 6th book of Mahabharata). The Gita narrates the dialogue between prince Arjuna and his guide and charioteer Lord Krishna in the search for liberation. I know it is sometimes difficult to read mythological books from different cultures as we are not accustomed to names and traditions. However, the teaching in human nature and our turmoil of emotions is universal.

Through the Gita and the genealogical tree of emotions we can understand the causes of suffering in our human existence. The intricate relationship between love and fear and their progeniture reveals a tapestry of entangled threads that change the picture and colours according to the degree of the internal dialogue.

Semantics

The Oxford dictionary definition of semantic is:

The branch of linguistics and logic concerned with meaning. The two main areas are logical semantics, concerned with matters such as sense and reference and presupposition and implication, and lexical semantics, concerned with the analysis of word meanings and relations between them.

Logical and Lexical. In sum, how we interact with a word and its mental meaning and how they marry together.

How do we think? Where does the information come from? What do we value as knowledge and truth? How does this affect our behaviour, our body our mental, physical and emotional health?

Is there a universal intelligence that we derive from that we tap into with the purpose to get information?

One day I was talking to Abhilash who is one of my clients, and it occurred to me the following analogy.

We, as humans, can only hear a certain range of frequencies and we can only see a range of vibrational waves therefore we may have a partial sense of reality triggered by semantics.

Abhilash is a mathematician, a programmer of artificial intelligence so I had to create a language limited by my short knowledge of this field. However, with some lexica we could communicate with each other.

I said: Imagine that we consider our reality, our entire universe, our collective consciousness's creation of science, religion, metaphysics, any level of cultural belief, and perception from any sense, was a designed programme based on predetermined parameters. Everything we think as reality, subconscious thoughts, conscious ones; everything we know, we see, we perceive, any named thing, unknown one is there. Imagine that any imaginable thought can pass your mind is a pixel in your programme. An equation where start and finish are axioms. The protocols to generate your programme are based on a binary system, 1 and 0, where 1 and 0 can be your own self. After all, we are the biological product of 2 separated entities, a Y and an X and we live in a reality of duality.

Your programme can evolve and trigger new updates in the collective consciousness, however, the range of expansion is pre-determined by the capability to create mental concepts that are named. If you can name it, it does exist. Existence in our reality becomes an entity when there is a symbiotic semantic.

You cannot imagine what you cannot perceive, and when you perceive it you name it. Even the unimaginable is a creation as it has a name. Its name is a negation of its opposite but as such it exists, it is like -1 exists as the negation of 1.

Does this mean that there are other universes, other realities parallel to our own reality? Yes and no. The logic will determine that the answer is yes, if in our reality consciousness exists why should it not exist anywhere else, after all, dogs can hear frequencies we cannot hear and other animals can see what we cannot see. We created machines to hear and to see what we cannot so why should there not be another perception of my own self somewhere else? Or not?

I have some clients who have been diagnosed with mental disorders and they have what we call hallucinations and have the perception of other realities, are they really ill or do they just have the ability to see what we cannot see?

Any explanation, any science, any concept and visual experimentation, observation, methodology, any scientific process cannot go beyond the mental process of the observer who has created it.

We can have responses which can be inconclusive, unknown, undetermined but even these answers are something!

Human evolution is based on the ability to communicate internal dialogues and create a collective consciousness. We have seen that scientific discoveries or inventions may happen in two different countries at the same time. Different individuals have come across with new understandings and their semantics.

Time to time we have individuals so unique that trigger new concepts and understanding, an exponential expansion in our parameters of reality. They can be in any field; Spiritually, to me, Jesus and Buddha convey a wonderful message of liberation through unconditional love. Their teachings can be as light or as profound according to their audience.

Quantum physics and quantum mechanics are fascinating not only by expanding our understanding of the collective but philosophically speaking it can help in the understanding of our inner dialogues. It is the simplification of the communion of the self with the universe, where everything is possible.

We are all energy, we resonate and vibrate, we have a frequency and we have developed a consciousness of a created reality in pursuance of creating awareness of our own self. How can an entity that does not differentiate itself have conscious knowledge of its existence without a contrast? We create the world where we live, we have evolved to compare and to name!

To give you an example, how much we validate concepts are related to the assumption of what it is truth or myth. Religion is a fantastic creation which provides a different lexicon to any phenomena that science will try to demonstrate is absurd. In reality, most of the time the same things are named with different names.

The creation of the world and the Bible. Six days God took to create the world... Definition of a day may vary. A day in a cosmic almanac can take billions of years.

In the beginning was darkness and chaos, God had created the Universe but it was unshaped. Then there was light and order.

The Big Bang theory in poetry! An explosion of energy that generates light.

Then there was expansion and creation of the planets, formation of heaven and earth. Day and night.

It sounds to me like the explanation of the formation of the atmosphere, dissipation of gases, creation of the moon as a satellite of the Earth.

It was creation of lands and oceans, again, creation of continents and volcanic activity that shifted tectonics plates and land and waters became separated.

Then there was the creation of plants, trees and seeds and God saw good in that. Also, the distinction between day and night. As soon atmosphere was created and photosynthesis started the skies were cleared, perhaps after all the volcanic activity had ceased and the clouds of fumes had settled down there was more distinction between day light and darkness, I do not know for sure as I was not there.

Then God said: "Let the waters swarm with living creatures, and let flying creatures fly above the earth across the expanse of the heavens.

Accordingly, to scientific study, animal life started in the sea, then evolved onto land and then there was the evolution of birds.

Then God said: "Let the earth bring forth living creatures according to their kinds, domestic animals and creeping animals and wild animals of the earth"

We know by evolutionary studies that Mammals were later in the evolution after amphibians, reptiles and birds.

Then he created men to populate and dominate the Earth! What a mistake! Then God took a rest.

Again, evolution taught us that homo sapiens were the last species to appear.

So, the explanations are similar it is just the semantics that change. The most important thing is that the world is created by a verbal command; God says!

An act of creation through verbalizing a mental concept. We cannot conceive a God manifesting matter without the use of words.

Also, there is the implication that creation came from a vibration, a sound from a voice, a conscious intention that transformed energy through a mental process.

When I was a teenager I spent many hours reading the Classics of Greek Philosophy. I adored Socrates and I fought the Sophists alongside him and I had imagined befriending the pre-Socratic scholars who had the most brilliant ideas about the origin of things and nature. I was fascinated by these men who were expressing their beautiful concepts in the 500s BC.

A few concepts are still in the background of my mind. Take Anaximandro of Mileto (547 A. C.). The principle of matter is ápeiron (unidentify, limitless, with no definition): The undetermined that is immortal, omnipotent and infinite.

He also talks about opposites as essential in the understanding of the evolution. This concept is later taken by Heráclito, Parménides, Empédocles and followers of Pitagoras.

He also believed in the existence of infinite worlds; different realities manifested in other universes.

Heráclitus of Éfeso (500 A. C.). He believed in the transformational fluidity and constant movement that creates contrast. All flows, all becoming.

Reality is composed of contraries; whose continual process of change is precisely what keeps it at rest.

You cannot bath twice in the same river as the water is not the same and you are also not the same.

He describes ignorance as the lack of genuine understanding. He speaks of a "logos" (translatable as "word," "rationality," "language," "ratio," and so forth) that most people do not understand.

Many are asleep, despite being awake. "Having heard without comprehension, they are like the deaf; this saying bears witness to them: present they are absent".

Most people do not observe the world carefully, and few attain a true understanding of it.

There is in Heraclitus a distinction between possessing data and understanding of how all of it fits together, what it all means, that is, its overall significance.

Perhaps, the concept of God, for Heraclitus, is synonymous with reality, so that a real understanding of the universe is an understanding of what is sacred. God is "day-night, winter-summer, war-peace", a unity of opposites.

Empedocles of Acragas (495 BC) was the first to name the four elements as earth, air, fire, and water. He also believed there were two forces that controlled and manipulated the elements; these forces were Love as the force that brings these elements in harmony, and the things generated from them, together, while Strife rives them. Empedocles repeatedly refers to a ceaseless cycle of unity from plurality a movement of Love, in unity with a movement of Strife.

Love and Strife are neutral terms, just opposite forces with no moral connotation; simply the natural forces regulated by universal laws that guide the ceaseless motion of being.

Plato and I spent hours together; his myth of the cavern and his explanation of how the soul falls into the body and the concept of reality was so real to me. I love him in a very platonic way!

I interpreted his concept that we are in a cavern and we just can see the reflection of the light in the opposite wall, light that comes from a small crack on the wall like a projector in a theatre and the film was what we could understand as a reality.

For several years, in my meditation I was pushing my brain to create expanded concepts of reality. One exercise that I used to do was to imagine I was in Plato's cavern and I had put on different stands, artefacts with a designed circle in the middle filled with a coloured glass. They were in line between myself and the crack in the cavern.

After Plato, the light was so intense that if we turned and looked at the light we could get blind and we were not able to cope with the pure source of light, like Icarus we would melt our wax wings if we get to close to the sun.

My logic determined that if I was gradually turning and looking to the light through my different coloured glasses and taught my eyes to perceive new lights I could eventually, get closer to the reality and its inner truth.

My perception of reality indeed changed as I was aware of my own capabilities to expand.

The point here is not how much I enjoyed the Greek company but the inner dialogues, my own semantics.

Which is your semantic? What is the dialogue that your mind is communicating to your brain?

In Buddhism, there is an analogy with darts. Your mind is constantly bombarding you with darts that cause you harm. They come in waves and most of the time they put you down and make you feel in doubt of yourself and create fears and misery.

Circumstances throw to you two darts of suffering, one is the physical pain that we undergo as a natural reaction or alert to danger, as the sensation we get when we burn ourselves and so on. Then, there is the mental suffering that little "evil" voice we hear that hurts us in a different way.

Buddha refers to the perception of feelings. Anyone can have pleasant ones, painful and neutral feelings. A trained disciple can have pleasant ones, painful and neutral feelings. Good, bad and neutral in any aspect in life we are confronted with these emotions. Now, where is the difference? And Buddha explains that it is our reaction and the attachment to the pleasure, resistance to pain or ignorance to our neutral emotions that makes the difference.

For those not trained, they get attached to sensual pleasure and seek pleasure as a remedy to pain. When he/she is touched by a painful (bodily) feeling, he worries and grieves, he laments, weeps and is distraught. He thus experiences two kinds of feelings, a bodily and a mental feeling. It is as if a man were pierced by a dart and, following the first piercing, he is hit by a second one.

For those who create a resistance and resent it experience two types of pain a bodily and a mental feeling and that emotions start to undermine their minds. Under the impact of that painful feeling they seek to escape from it through the enjoyment of sensual pleasure. Sensual happiness is the only mechanism they know to escape instead of embracing and facing their own pain. Honour the purpose of its existence and do not be in denial or resist. As the resistance grows it creates a weakness in the mind. It is like being hit twice, creating patterns that sedate and numb your mind but still creating an underlying condition.

We can experience any dart, the first one we cannot avoid; however, we can see it for what it is and we can master our reaction. Feel the pain, experience it and release it. There is no need to seek an escape route and compensate with pleasure as sooner or later it will hit us.

Set your mind free and face circumstances as they come, regardless of the arising and ending of the feelings, nor the gratification, the danger and the escape, connected with them.

I was with my client Helen and she told me she was having anxiety issues. She suddenly had panic attacks and she did not even know why. She told me that she gets very scared even when she is in familiar environments, at home, in the street, anywhere.

She did not know why this was happening to her or how to deal with it.

I created a scenario for her. I told her to imagine a theatre. I told her she was the director of a well-produced company and she was creating a play. The tone of the play was up to her; as a director, she had the power to produce any play of her liking.

Some scenes could be very dramatic with a climax and then some cathartic release. She could add some comedy or a post-modern style of pure realism and even a hint of the absurd. Because it is your life, how much drama or melodrama she puts into it is her choice and right. As the director, she has the power to determine her own play. I wanted her to see her own play as a spectator and create a target audience (her own self), where she could study their reaction. I said "their" and not her as we have many different characters acting in a play and many sides of us observing the play. The intensity of drama in our life is up to us, it is our own reaction to stimulus. It is our internal monologue that writes the script. Now; how to play it is up to us.

When you write your own play, study your characters diligently, observe them, identify their nuances, their background, go deep into them with the wonderful disposition of being a creator and not a victim of your own drama. That inner dialogue must be a tool for the artist and not the other way around.

And remember it is a play, a scenario of your own creation. Empower yourself to become your own director.

I noticed that when my clients leave me they are free of pain, free of mental issues and then a few days later they fall into the same learned process from their past.

It is very difficult to break with learned patterns of behaviour. Our brain has created routes like motorways that trigger an automated response taking you in the direction that you are used to. It is like turning in the wrong exit as we used to live somewhere else.

The human process of learning and understanding is divided in different phases.

At first, we are completely oblivious of our own ignorance living in a state of unconscious ignorance; and then we are aware of our ignorance until we reach a conscious understanding of knowledge aiming to achieve an unconscious level of knowledge.

When we do things as second nature, automating a process, we have really absorbed the information creating new paths of neurotransmitters, nonetheless we need repetition and belief and focus in the new pathway to create a permanent link to the transmission.

Perseverance is the key and that can only happen when you realise you love yourself and it is worth to work for a happier you.

When we realise that we live a life in ignorance, we are demoralised as our ego starts judging us and feeling that we were happier in ignorant bliss. We have the choice to give up and deny our self-discovery, and carry on as usual while undermining the mind with more pain.

The problem is that there is point of non-return, when we start a journey of self-realization. It is like you have a glance to the light directly from the crack in the cavern and you cannot take that image away from your eyes.

Another aspect you need to take into consideration is integrity and honesty to yourself. We cannot jump steps, we have to do a profound introspective journey, not leaving any rock unturned. Be honest to your own self, with love and compassion.

Sometimes I have clients who come with deep emotional pain, that they have masked and their body so kindly has stored for them at the peril to get ill itself, waiting for the time that the person is ready to release that energy.

When I get in contact with that energy information starts emanating, flashes of images that the body stored like the file name in the archive. We can store these files everywhere in the body, so many times we heard doctors dismissing a condition because it is "psychosomatic" "It is all in your mind" they said. The news is everything is in the mind.

We are energy manifested as matter, we vibrate at a range of frequencies that our conception of reality interprets as matter through the semantic dialogue between brain and mind.

Our emotions are energy, that resonate at different frequencies. Positive emotions are promoting relaxation, homeostasis (balance, equilibrium), that requires less energy to flow. There are energy savers as they are smooth and just flow synergistically with the Universe.

Negative emotions need to be dealt with. In the same way that our immune system deals with foreign bodies and harmful microorganisms, our emotional receptors deal with negativity.

We shield our emotions and store them and use a lot of energy and resources to perform. We create hormones that trigger stress responses. We use antioxidants and nutrients to counter the oxidative processes and the release of free radicals; our metabolism changes and all our physiognomy pays the price.

The energy we stored gets stagnant and trapped. We ignore the meaning of the original message brought by the first dart and distort it which keeps the wound bleeding. We put it in the drawer of oblivion and then carry on undeterred by the damage of its toxicity. Toxicity that will be diffused through a root system touching other aspects of your life.

There are two fields of master emotions from where all the other emotions emerge. These emotions are love and fear.

In our binary system where existence is based on opposites, we have these two juxtaposed forces.

Fear is the base of creation of life's lessons. Fear is the mother of all questions while Love has only answers.

Fear of not having enough triggers greed, envy, jealousy, anxiety, selfishness, self-centred, despotic, manipulative, pride, sense of poverty, inferiority, sense of not being good enough, competitiveness, skepticism, lack of deservedness amongst other things you can think of.

It also triggers violence, aggression, anger, dishonesty, hate, heaviness, pessimism, sadness, criticism, contemptuousness, victimization, blaming others, resentfulness, and all the lacks you can imagine. Lack of love, lack of money, lack of success, lack of health.

Love is the solution. Love is the repairer, the binder that neutralises the fear. From Love, we feel compassion, kindness, generosity, forgiveness, humility, respectful of self and others, awareness of our own achievements, sense of responsibility, honesty, integrity, happiness, optimism, inspirational, altruism, good sense of humour and many others you can imagine giving you a good feeling.

The key is that when you think about it you find yourself with a smile on your face and a feeling of release on your chest.

It is up to you to realise in which field you want to be. Sometimes we enjoy putting ourselves in the fear camp as it is easier. How great is blaming others and circumstances and weather and ancestors, and culture and KARMA!!!

Karma, sin, punishment, retribution… What are they?

They are opportunities, just an act that teaches us to do things differently in order to get a less painful experience next time.

Karma is not a punishment, as sin is not an act against God.

Karma is a process to realise what our unconsciousness is trying to manifest in our conscious reality. Lessons we need to experience to release obstacles that hinder our understanding of happiness.

Karma is another mechanism to empty unfinished emotional developments that we perceive as good or bad in a social moral frame.

We are ruled by universal laws, one of them is cause and effect.

For every action, there is an equal and opposite reaction; for every effect, there is a definite cause, likewise for every cause, there is a definite effect.

Your thoughts, behaviours and actions create specific effects that manifest and create your life as you know it.

My clients arrive and they tell me they have problems, problems, problems…. I simply said good! That sounds great, as problems are simply manifestations of a specific input that brought an undesired outcome.

See your problem as an opportunity to expand, to create new avenues, to trigger new input and to detach from the outcome.

A solution is only a different outcome!

We cannot lie to our own soul. The universe flows in truth. No matter what we do, we will always have an opportunity to flow in synchronicity with a universal opus that flows effortlessly in a melody where all is truth. Energy expands and flows in harmony. Truth is harmony, is diaphanous, like pure crystalline water running seamlessly that compels you to love and relax.

Problems are just manifestations that produce a resistance to your own truth. More resistance more blockages are manifested to show you that your flow has taken a secondary course where you need a higher input of energy to go across.

The greater the input of energy the pricier for your own health it is. More resistance also will involve more mental dialogue that would create more pollution that sooner or later creates disease.

The inner dialogue that can exacerbate your perception of reality. Also, your semantics, be aware of the way you talk. Your language is important.

You manifest your verb! Syntax is a great science. When you decompose a sentence you realise that each word has a power. Each word is like an embryo which has its own energetic value and position. Intention and strength are expressed to words and communication through sentences, sentences to paragraphs and when you see it is the volumes of your life story.

Whatever you say (inner dialogue or verbally expressed by your voice, image or writing) your brain will interpret as a truth, it will generate a belief.

To give you an example, swearing, I always said to Drew not to swear in vain, as each opprobrium vituperation has an energetic charge that is higher than regular language. An input in the word that involves an emotional reaction. Anger, pain, fear, hate, aggression, besmear, love, empathy, kindness, anything can be expressed by words, all of them have an energetic charge that produce a reaction, so, be kind to yourself and use language as a tool and not as a weapon.

Remember that your neurons have the ability to create new paths of communication conveying new ideas that can create new truths that will minimise the input of energy therefore dissipating resistance. You will be able to embrace the circumstances of daily life without generating high levels of stress.

The process of communication from cell to cell is call synapsis, they jump from cell to cell, a conceived idea triggers electrical charges that send messages to different areas of your body. In the endocrine system, they trigger a release of messengers that triggers the production of hormones.

Stress hormones will act in all the metabolic and physiological functions in your body, creating a boost of input of energy that needs to be counterbalanced to reduce the wear you have generated.

How are you feeling now? Do you need a break? Perhaps a cup of tea?

Have a little break and we can continue later...

But before you leave, I will try, in my ill manner to tell you a joke. I am terrible at telling jokes. I even found jokes funny that are terrible!

I am witty and I love laughing. I love being happy and find life light and not too serious. I may say, I consider myself with a great sense of humour, but it is so difficult to show it while writing about neuroplasticity.

Here it goes:

Why did the cows leave the field on Sunday nights?

To go to the MOOOOvies...

I told you it was terrible!

See you later...

Detachment

What is this word all about? De-attachment.

Is it to become cold, unsensitive, careless? Is it to go to live in a monastery, disconnected from the mundane world? Is it poverty? Is it to renounce your family, material possessions, money, work, sex, fun?

Is this a religious, mystical, mumbo jumbo stuff? A New Era, hippy talk? The good thing is that it is none of the above.

Detachment is a liberation, it is freedom from pain and suffering. It is unconditional love. Think about our own children. We want them to be happy, independent, we raised them to become their own persona.

We are caretakers of these young lives and we want them to leave our side and create their own families and prosper in every aspect. We want to see a part of us in them; to see a reflection of the input that we made the best we could.

We love them therefore, we let them fly away in their own right. We would be there for them when they need us. Our creations have become creators and we must step aside. That is detachment. To love with no attachments, like every day is our own creation and whatever is in it has the same right to exist without one claiming ownership.

We do not own our children, and any creation of us, is one's child.

If we do not own flesh that was created in our entrails, flesh that share one's inner imprint we do not own anything else.

It is like the artist creator of a piece that it is not complete until it transcends as art when it stops belonging to the artist and encounters the spectator; the artist as creator is transformed by its creation while learning to let it go. His art will transcend his own existence and will become his legacy, a name; a Da Vinci, a Picasso, it is no longer the flesh and blood it is the canvas and the oils that transcends.

Sometimes we are attached to pain. It is easier to live in fear, in perpetuating the torment as it is familiar, it is continuity and cautiousness.

It is easier to suffer than to confront the root of the attachment and release it... change involves a mourning of the past and anxiety of what is to come.

However, being detached is liberating and virtuous. It brings you inner peace as it generates a sense of respect not only to others, (things, animals, people) but to yourself.

It brings integrity, honesty, comfort, happiness, humility and self-confidence as it does not allow fear to exist.

There is no fear of not having enough, or fear to lose what we have, fear of being rejected, abandoned.

Ownership does not really exist. When we buy a car, we exchanged two different energies. We give money (that it is indeed a source of energy materialised in a concept that allows an exchange of matter) in exchange of a designed structure composed of metal, plastic, etc. that travels.

That we extend our name to objects is a practical method to make us responsible for the object in question.

As you see, when you buy a car it is in your name; in your name to pay taxes, insurance, to identify it from others.

We work for a determined period of time and in exchange we get a figure of numbers deposited in a bank account. That figure becomes closer to the concept of money when we exchange it for a service or goods.

Money is an energy that we do not own. By definition, it has to flow, to be circulated and exchanged to be transformed into objects. Your £5 note is per se a piece of plastic, just when you go to the café it becomes a latte. When you give that note to the barrister it becomes money then it is put in the cash register where it becomes a piece of plastic. The synergy triggers the concept of value.

Then the café owner, counts the notes, takes them to the bank, deposits it in his account, the bank makes a record of his input, puts the notes in the ATM and then you go and withdraw from the machine and the cycle starts again.

Money is not evil, it triggers fears when there is not detachment. The energy of money has to circulate otherwise it becomes stagnant rotten waters. Greed is stagnation, the desire of amassing regardless how much we have is a fear of not having enough.

When money does not circulate, inequality happens, the richer become richer and the poor become poorer and the class in the middle gets overstretched, pushed downwards and fighting to keep the neck above the water as the last effort before drowning into the abyss.

Then, not content to do this to each other we do it to the planet. We destroy nature every day, we rob her from her little treasures that she already so generously gives to us. Multinational corporations become anonymous, faceless, monsters that proliferate like cancers feeding their tumorous stockholders to satiate their thirst of greed.

We see the destruction of the rain forest, the natural habitats of other species, pollution of waters and contamination with heavy metals and toxic waste from different industries. Just to name one example, in Colombia a natural pristine forest was destroyed with the contamination of Mercury and other heavy metals as consequence of the mining industry extracting gold in the region. Fauna and flora destroyed, waters contaminated, fish dying, plants dying, mammals, birds all of them dying; humans with tumours and malformed fetuses with mutations and then they do not count as they do not have any influence, no voice, no value. Their aboriginal hamlets are poor and isolated.

Global warming, despite the skepticism of the oil industry and their figurehead Donald Trump, exists. The hoax is their tongues, how can they contradict the laws of physics regarding matter, that it cannot be created or destroyed, just transformed? The burning of fossil oils has to transform into something. The transformation into energy, into heat, movement, electricity creates sub products and those gases have to go somewhere. Some of them are absorbed and processed by plants, get fixed in the oceans in the atmosphere and their presence create a chemical transformation that will affect the environment. For every cause, there is a reaction, for every CO_2 emissions the Ph in the Ocean will get acidic, with acidity the coral will die, banks of fish and plants will disappear.

How can it be possible that we do not honour life in all its splendour while seeing magnificent creatures like elephants destroyed for their fangs just to make decorative useless objects! Taking a life for nothing! And then sharks killed for their dorsal fins to make a soup!

Rhinoceros for their horns for sexual arousal and folkloric medicinal beliefs of transferring stamina and strength, while we are transforming a life into a carcass.

Life is the most beautiful treasure we have, life force is our essence, our energy, our divine intelligence. Only love, gratitude, detachment can emerge from it.

We are all linked, we are all share the same origin, we are all facing the same consequences of any action, that it is the principle of the butterfly flaps its wings in the other side of the planet and somewhere it will have an effect.

By destroying the planet, we destroy ourselves, a portion of our unconditional love suffers, our soul sobs, as we are all a manifestation of that segment of collective consciousness we call reality.

Do not get me wrong, I do appreciate beautiful, high quality things. Not for the monetary value or status, I just like to honour the craftsmanship, the thought, passion, integrity, respect and dedication behind the conceived object. I am happy to know that all the individuals who participated in that creation got remunerated accordingly; however, how many of those we things do we really need? How much do we depend on the symbols of prosperity to feel superior, better or richer? How many of those things does a person require and to what extent are these objects influencing our emotions? How happy are you by possessing these objects and how miserable do you will feel when someone takes them away? How many of these things can we happily give away and help those who are in need?

And then, it is not only objects, it is the way we look, the products we use to stop the passing of time, the perception of how others see us, the images we portray, what we say, the people who are around us.

So, detachment is not being outside of the world, it is not being unsensitive and careless, quite the opposite, it is realising the sense of belonging in the sense of being part of a whole, in union, as equals. It is being aware of "to be".

Buddha talks about detachment, he even warns us regarding escaping to a monastery and abandoning the world. He says to be aware of your own ego as by living a monastic life may you think you are more noble than others, that you are better as you can set yourself free from materialism, by judgement of yourself and others, you are in fact carrying a bigger attachment.

So, whatever is your lifestyle, in the monastery or outside of it, just be aware of the freedom of non-ownership, imagine the responsibility! Being accountable of every breath you take! Boring!

One way of being detached is by being mindful. Honour and value every interaction in your life. Each minute as it was your last, just enjoy and interact.

The same happens when we love someone, when we are romantically involved with some other being. We confuse love as an exchange of energy that we entitle ownership upon it.

We do not own the person. They do not own us, or even better we do not owe them anything and they do not owe anything either.

Two beings felt love for each other. Two equals became connected, intrinsic part of a union but there is not ownership. For how long? Who knows and it is not really important. It can last until the end of their lives or not. It does not matter.

Mr. Trump wanted to redecorate the White House, as now, it must be gilded, tacky and flashy.

So, he decided to get three quotes. The first one came from a group of illegal immigrants who told him. "Mr. Trump, we will do the job for 1 million dollars, the thousands of us who are from Mexico, Nicaragua, San Salvador, Honduras, but to make it easier for you call us Mexicans, we will do the painting, the decoration and for free we will do the landscaping and the cleaning".

Then the American team came and told him, "Mr. Trump we will do it for 7 million dollars with three coats of high quality paint".

Then it came the Colombian one, who said, "Mr. Trump, I will do it for 10 million dollars. 5 for me, 4 for you and we give one million to the Mexicans to do the job!"

Compartmentalisation of concepts

Our minds have the tendency to be tidy! Little compartments for everything and they cannot overlap, they cannot even touch.

It is like reasoning is the sum of little boxes. Everything based on contrast. One thing cannot be something else at the same time! Concepts, concepts, concepts! Limiting your creativity and your freedom.

Our conception of thoughts determines the expansion of our mind therefore our personality.

How apprehensive and cautious we are, our sense of humour, how seriously we take life, how good we are at taking decisions, how much we adapt, what we believe, what we love, etc.

We taint, we smear, we preconceive and we assume things even before we understand their nature.

We are so prompt to judge, to ridicule, to discard and to discredit what we do not feel comfortable with.

We are like knights in bright armor riding a white horse defending with honour our assumptions, our maximum degree of tolerance is to agree to disagree.

To give you an example, take the dialectical method.

Dialectical method is the use of reasoning to resolve disagreement through rational discussion, and, ultimately, the search for truth.

Socrates was passionate about this method, as for him it was essential to postulate an hypothesis, then through reasoning and not rhetoric, the proposal of an antithesis that leads to a contradiction; thus, forcing arguments to validate both sides in search for the truth.

In modern Philosophy, we adapted a method based on the triad of thesis, antithesis, synthesis often used to describe the thought of German philosopher Georg Wilhelm Friedrich Hegel, despite that Hegel never used the term himself. For Hegel, the concrete, the synthesis, the absolute, must always pass through the phase of the negative, in the journey to completion, that is, mediation.

The Hegelian dialectic consist of:

1. Thesis (abstract, that it is the initial proposition)

2. A negation of that thesis called the antithesis (negative)

3. Synthesis (Concrete), that it is a compromise of the above, a new proposition that can start the process again.

So, think of White as the Thesis, then Black as the Antithesis and Grey as the synthesis, however, it does not take into consideration the shades of grey if there are 50 or more! It is after all, only a grey area!

What it is interesting in Hegel's point of view is that he takes into consideration the concept of unity. We need to embrace our opposite to determine the truth. Embrace what we negate, what makes us uncomfortable to set us free of judgment. After all, we are a nuance of shades of whites and blacks; we do not know exactly when a dirty white becomes grey, how much black we need to add in order to transform the white into charcoal and how much white we need to eliminate in the charcoal to call it pitch black.

We all deserve to be here and to be happy and fulfilled. We all deserve to love and to be loved and have the deep knowledge that love is there for us independently of us doing our best or not.

We have to learn to detach ourselves from the mentality of reward. If I do something for you, you will do something for me, and so on, not only with people but with things, circumstances, at home, at work, everywhere.

We do not need to be good or bad, one just needs to be. Goodness, kindness as any other emotion has to emanate effortlessly, innocently and spontaneously with no expectations.

They are natural manifestations like breathing, sleeping, eating. So, why are you waiting for a reward, feeling good with yourself, for approval, for compensation?

The attachment to recognition is painful and weakens you as your happiness and self-value depends on a gesture coming from others.

We do not have to do something to trigger a result. When one understands this, enters in the process called Enlightment, a liberation from cause and effect.

When you reach that Eureka moment, you are in the process of Self-Realization.

Self-Realization is simply the ability to observe the inner self manifested with no filters, untainted by life experiences, egos, cultural knowledge, etc.

It is the freedom to be, just being! Understanding, comprehension and wisdom comes when they are needed, otherwise living in a space of nothingness.

It is the realization that emptiness is a bliss and being nothing is the pure form of existence, where all the opposites become one, become nothing. A space where your mind is quiet.

It is the underline feeling that you are part of the whole, like being a particle of a DNA sequence in the Universe's genome.

It feels like an extension of a greater order or intelligence. You may call it God, Divine, Cosmic, Force, Intelligence, the name after all is part of semantics. It is perhaps the concept that it is nameless as you can feel it but escapes the mind's ability to describe it.

In the Chakra system, there are two whirlpools corresponding to your ego or identification of the self.

One of them is the Hrit Padma that it is around two fingers below your heart and the second one named Manipura or Solar Plexus.

Hrit Padma in the Yogic tradition corresponds to the pure heart, the spiritual heart that is the essential and ultimate transcendent consciousness of one's being.

It is another name for the Supreme Self, or Atman. The Spiritual Heart is the Supreme Consciousness, the ultimate subject of knowledge, the pure I. It is the observer, the witness of unfolding existence. That intimate observer of all our thoughts, emotions and sensations; the witness of both, the mind and the universe in its inner and outer dimensions.

It is where the knowledge and differentiation of that Universal being resides.

Manipura, is the conscious self as separated entity, the you, the I, that makes as different from anyone else. It is the ego that identifies us with our judgements, perceptions, emotions, thoughts and so and so.

Manipura is located behind the navel. The Manipura Chakra contains many precious jewels such as the qualities of clarity, self-confidence, bliss, self-assurance, knowledge, wisdom and the ability to make correct decisions.

So, in sum, we have two egos the big one at soul level the universal one, and the little one who rules our reality.

When the third chakra (Solar Plexus) is closed, we may feel tired, afraid, withdrawn. There is a fear of taking risks, confronting people or issues, taking charge, being judgmental and putting ourselves down. We doubt ourselves and have the tendency towards self-judgement, comparing, copying and complying with the masses.

You will find issues about fear of rejection, and being overly concerned with what others can think about you. You may be highly sensitive to criticism with very low self-esteem, self-confidence and self-respect.

A blocked Solar Plexus will generate feelings of insecurity, fear of being alone, with the need of constant reassurance.

You may avoid responsibility, decision making and have issues around trust and personal honour.

There may be too much seriousness and rigidity with not enough laughter, ease, or fun, all of which help the third chakra to open and relax.

If the Chakra is too open, then we have a kind of bully archetype personality who always needs to be in control, to dominate, to seek power, prestige, ambition.

Individuals with an overactive chakra have the tendency to be aggressive, over controlling, workaholics, judgmental, deep anger, who like to rule through fear and intimidation.

As the tendency of these characters are more ego orientated, they can become narcissistic and self-centred.

An appropriate countermeasure to help balancing this chakra is the concept of the warrior-standing strong archetype, staying in touch with your feelings, confronting only when appropriate, and quietly maintaining a sense of power.

A robust Solar plexus can take on tasks and complete them, take on risks and not be bound by perfectionism. It can act in the role of leadership without domination or self-ennoblement.

Suppressed anger and depression are the psychological obstacles of this chakra.

This chakra is also teaching us a need to apologise and to forgive not only others but most importantly one's self.

We can learn to release the inner critic from limiting belief patterns and self-sabotaging behaviour by positive intentions and setting healthy goals triggering lifestyles changes.

So, from now on, please laugh a little bit more and take yourself less seriously, relax and enjoy. Life is beautiful!

Why do we have the need to judge?

Why we must value the concept of "ours" as better than others? In which mental process, we determine that in order to appreciate something we have to put others down. It is like intrinsic value does not count by itself.

We need to compare and assess. To analyse and determine on which side of the seesaw we will sit.

We need to compete and strive and take sides. We give a judgment and we put it in a scale of values. From one extreme to another. Whatever characteristics we like we assimilate them, we display them, we claim ownership over them and we argue with other groups over who had it first!

Suddenly to become "Numero UNO" is king! War, death, destruction, annihilation of cultures, beliefs, territories, nature; all is justified in the pursuit of our interests.

Going from one extreme to another, like in a park playing on a seesaw. The one down, is putting the power, to root one's self, to validate his superiority, to put weight in his statements.

The one up, the de-rooted one, is at the mercy of his opponent but putting resistance until the other gives up due to tiredness or boredom.

Then the roles reverse, a new reign starts until it gives up. Ephemeral ups and downs as a reflection of their own selves. No one is interested being in harmony, right in the middle both contenders holding the same weight, in equilibrium, in a state of contemplation. We will not be able to hold that position for long as we get distracted and we decide that it is boring and we go...

We have the park of History to see the ups and downs; they come and go like a pendulum in perfect symmetry. We can see it in Art History, when we think of art as a cultural manifestation that reflects the mental/emotional state of their individuals; different currents in contradistinction to the next movement.

From Classicism to Mediaeval. Then from Renaissance to Baroque. Next, the pendulum swings back and forth, from Baroque to the opposite; the Neoclassical. Again, it moves to Romanticism, and in response to it, we have Realism, then Impressionism. Born in response to the impressionist there it comes the Post-Impressionism, then Fauvism, etcetera.... etcetera...

It seems we have to deny an idea in order to validate a second one. Exclusion instead of inclusion. Separation and judgment instead of integration and acceptance.

Once, I had a new client. He came for a massage and we were chatting. He had his treatment and we carried on talking for a short while. He was most agreeable and perhaps thought to pay a compliment and then he said:

"You are pretty clever for a masseuse". To what I replied: "Oh, thank you, I am so grateful, how kind of you. Sorry, I do not want to sound ungrateful; it seems a little bit discriminatory, you see; intelligent people have the right to work with their hands too!".

Intelligence, Science, Religion, Spirituality, the same difference?

Why do we associate Intelligence with Science?

And, why do we separate it from Religion or Spirituality?

And even, why do we associate Religion with Spirituality?

Are they not part of a whole? Is their interpretation not a product of the mind and communicated verbally or graphically with others?

Why cannot we associate Intelligence to Spirituality?

Where is the boundary? In our ego? Again, is this a need to understand and compartmentalise concepts of pseudo-opposites?

Why do they need to be antagonistic? How can we associate them and accept them as part of the spectrum of energy we conceive as reality?

If we part from the axiom that what we consider real extends up to the capabilities of our brain to comprehend and our mind to interpret; everything has the same origin, all emanates from the same intelligence and the process of their existence is through a mental process.

Why do we have to expel one in favour to the other? At the end, it is just a manifestation that differs from another with the purpose to provide guidance.

So, why in order to validate our arguments do we have to tarnish others?

We have the right to believe in whatever we want and to follow whatever path we want without the need to obscure others.

There is an intrinsic science behind any reasoning. A scientific process is based on observation, comparison, corroboration and conclusion.

We determine something is when it is not something else. When you have a hypothesis, in order to demonstrate it is valid, it needs to undergo a process that we have already validated as acceptable. If the object matter to demonstrate undergoes on the pre-approved process the results of the conclusion will be consider as truth.

The results of this conclusion can be a negative statement, can be inconclusive, can be a positive affirmation of what was initially searched to demonstrate. The conclusion is irrelevant if we understand and trust the logic in operation.

As long as there is congruency in the process the result becomes objective, a demonstrable truth, even if the postulate was false to start with!

And congruency comes from patterns in neurological connections that are articulated to review and recognize terms as familiar and tested bringing an outcome of approval or disapproval.

The brain will see it and say to itself: "Oh I recognise this I just have to connect it to the usual result so it must be truth!"

Rigour takes place in the process, we are like children designing the rules of a game.

In religion, the rules are different. They said to us, we have already proven the facts and you just need to believe us to be part of our team.

There was an initial guy who said wonderful things, we agreed with him and now we follow his thoughts. However, to do so, we need to create a set of rules, to make sure you really belong to this group. After all, despite the guy being a fantastic thinker and pushing us to see things differently and expand or consciousness we need to give it structure.

We need to make it bigger and more important, even better; give it a divine connection, after all it is so big, so important that it must come from a higher intelligence than ours.

Also, give it mysticism around to people to fear it and obey the word as it is the only way it will pass to posterity. We need to make money from it and build temples and impress others who will dare to compare our belief to theirs and decide that ours it is not at their level.

And then we create a collective and we create things around it and we expand its reality. Some of the initial thoughts are lost, misinterpreted, adapted, to the collective it serves it purpose. It does not mean it does not have validation or a purpose to exist.

Another game with another set of rules.

In all the religions that I have studied it seems to have a fundamental original universal truth that resonates with everyone regardless of your cultural, ethnic or geographical background.

Are all religions spiritual? Or is spirituality a religion?

Again, how many shades of grey we have in here. Can you be spiritual without being a religious person? The answer is yes!

For a moment think of Buddha and Jesus. They were not religious people per se but they were pivots of spirituality.

Buddha followed all the currents he found in his path; thought, sect, tradition, religion and nothing really satisfied him. There was something missing the emptiness, the knowing "that it was not it", feeling that he must go further, he just sat and found it deep in himself. Then he was fulfilled when reached that degree of emptiness and connected to that inner truth.

And what about Jesus who ended crucified by his compatriots. Jesus was a revolutionary, a multiplier of new ideas who not only converted fish and bread into thousands. He was the fisherman of men.

He started by preaching at the temple at 12, declaring himself the son of God, surrounded by fishermen, tax collectors, ladies of the night (allegedly), and anyone else who wanted to follow him. He destroyed the merchants organized bazaars at the temple. He questioned the patricians' ethics; he broke the rules and his cousin was baptizing people in the name of the Spirit submerging them under running waters.

Jesus was gaining momentum. He scared the establishment who eliminated him and his cousin John the Baptist.

Jesus knew the religion of his peers, he was a Jew himself; he knew the texts and he knew perhaps better than any other savant the interpretation of the scriptures. His vison was expanded, his knowledge was superior, his love was unconditional and yet he was not a Christian.

He died as a Jew; the Inri, IESVS·NAZARENVS·REX·IVDÆORVM (Iesus Nazarenus, Rex Iudaeorum), the "Jesus the Nazarene, king of Jews".

After him there were several martyrs, killed for following his ideas, thousands died during the Roman Empire until Constantine the Grand, in 313 AD, issued the Edict of Milan, officially legalizing Christian worship.

By then the Christian religion was already an organised one, under a structure of hierarchy. In the post-Apostolic church (after Jesus apostles had died around 100 AD), bishops emerged as overseers of urban Christian populations, and a hierarchy of clergy gradually took on the form of bishops, presbyters (priests), and then deacons (servants).

Sometimes when you put so many codes of conduct and restrictions, a religion loses its spirituality, it just comes a dogmatization of the masses, a tool for control instead of growth.

Spirituality relates more to an intimate connection between you and your inner self.

It relates to your own essence, to that cosmogonic transcended reality of the self. It is subtle as it is universal, it is intimate as it is global, it is your relationship to become one. It drives you to expand exponentially towards the consciousness of the universe by going to the deepest corners of your own soul.

It pushes you to create new semantics and awareness of unveiled neuroplastic connections ready to exist.

I would love to review other concepts with you that I consider important before we develop the IS Healing system.

Zen

The philosophical current of Zen is by definition, impossible to describe as by doing so, you lose the principle. As you see, the concept is to sever any logic pattern, a mental disruption to empty the mind; like breaking down neruoplastic connections, forcing the mind to change the semantics. To learn other type of dialogue, with no patterns, with no logic, with no purpose to confuse, to dissipate, to quieten the mind until it becomes silent.

However, by stating so, I am giving a logical explanation and a purpose to Zen, therefore my explanation is not valid even if the concept is in it; as it is stated logically it does not exist as Zen.

Everything started with Bodhidharma who was a Buddhist monk who lived during the 5th or 6th century. He is traditionally credited as the transmitter of Chan Buddhism or Zen to China. According to Chinese legend, he also began the physical training of the monks of Shaolin Monastery that led to the creation of Shaolin Kung Fu.

Zen Buddhism brings order in to chaos and has a very rich literature and long codes of practice based in Buddhism and meditation.

Bodhidharma's approach favoured the rejection of devotional rituals, doctrinal debates and verbal formalizations. He was inclined to an intuitive grasp of the "Buddha mind" within everyone, through meditation. Bodhidarma emphasized personal enlightenment, rather than the promise of heaven.

He also considered a holistic approach, spiritual, intellectual and physical excellence as an indivisible whole necessary for enlightenment.

Several stories about Bodhidharma have become popular legends, which are still being used in the Ch'an, Seon and Zen-tradition.

One such story is about an encounter with Emperor Xiao Yan

The Anthology of the Patriarchal Hall says that in 527, Bodhidharma visited Emperor Wu of Liang a fervent patron of Buddhism:

Emperor Wu: *"How much karmic merit have I earned for ordaining Buddhist monks, building monasteries, having sutras copied, and commissioning Buddha images?"*

Bodhidharma: *"None. Good deeds done with worldly intent bring good karma, but no merit."*

Emperor Wu: *"So what is the highest meaning of noble truth?"*

Bodhidharma: *"There is no noble truth, there is only emptiness."*

Emperor Wu: *"Then, who is standing before me?"*

Bodhidharma: *"I know not, Your Majesty."*

What is essential for us at this moment, it is the question of the Emperor, how much merit have I earned by doing so and so.

When we give a purpose, a reason to do something for a personal gain and not because is our natural state and there is no need of a reason, we are not evolving in a spiritual understanding.

People come to me asking what they need to do to improve their life. How can they be happier, what are the set of rules, what is the formula?

None. As long as you think life has a purpose greater than the one already intrinsic in itself; that life's purpose is life itself you will not understand it.

Sometimes people get upset with me as in social gatherings there is at least someone who comes and asks: "What do you do for a living" to which I reply: "I breath".

Integrity, honesty, pure, crystal, clear essence emanates from the soul when the mind is silent. There is not a purpose, a reason, an excuse. It just IS!

It is like asking what I need to do to have blue eyes when you are born with brown eyes. Apart of wearing fake contact lenses nothing, being blue eyed is not in your nature. But eyes are eyes and they have the ability to see.

Life's purpose is not to become a career, a job, a vocation. Married, single, parent or barren.

When we do good deeds, it is not for a recompense or to be appreciated or to be noticed by others, it is because, it is so in you that you do not even notice. It is your nature. It is your brown eyes or blue eyes.

When we say that person is so genuine, it is because we recognise an element of truth.

It is like giving to charity, to whom does it benefit more?

Jesus said that when you give with one hand the other hand should not know it. Otherwise; you are a Pharisee, a two-time masquerade gaining adulations by profiting on others suffering.

Be empty of an unseen agenda, be empty of a purpose and just enjoy life!

Tantra

If I should describe myself as a follower of a specific mentality, I would say that:

I am a Buddhist Tantrika who loves Jesus and enjoys Zen.

I am one who found useful concepts in the Gita as in the New Testament.

I am also the one who enjoys listening to Cox and loves watching the scientific programmes in the BBC4!

However, I do not label myself.

Every time that I speak about Tantra, I can hear the nervous giggles, and the cheeky, perky, youthful, eyes in people when their sweet ignorance makes them nervous and said Tantra and a silly laugh comes around and they whisper the Word, S E X, in small letters, SEX.

As if Tantra was related only to SEX or even if Tantra was synonymous to insidious debaucher! I found that very funny!

There is this book that I highly recommend if you want to go in a tantric journey. It is one of my favour books, it is The Tantra Experience, the Evolution through Love by Osho.

Osho talks about the integrative aspect of Tantra as it brings unity and acceptance through love. Tantra does not have the moral codes of good or bad that split your psyche. Tantra does not judge you, it just embraces you.

In Tantra, you reach states of freedom and joy as it does not have a cause and effect mandate, or a punishment; there is no guilt, nor shame, nor conflict. You are not judging yourself or others. There is not Heaven or Hell, not good or evil, it is only us, with all our emotions, with all our experiences, love, hate, fear, joy, anger, passion, desire, sex, jealousy, all of them and we recognise each one of them.

Things in life just are manifested, they are not a prize for good or bad behaviour.

Tantra is freedom of judgement. Tantra transubstantiates our existence. This transformation is possible when you accept your total being, then everything falls in place, the cause of our pain and suffering gets absorbed; anger, greed, fear, all of them are osmosed.

Tantra transforms but it does not condemn. All that is Devil can be seen as a seed of transformation. The Devil is trying to find the divine; there is an opportunity to become the Divine to evolve as a seed; its purpose is to become a tree and the tree to give fruit. The Divine is the tree fully in bloom and the Devil is the seed. The tree is hidden in the seed and the seed is not against the tree and the tree is not against the seed. They work in unison, in friendship. They are two phases of the same energy so are the contrast in life. Death and life, day and night, love and hate.

Osho explains the origin of Tantra. There are two currents one that came from Hinduism and the second one that derives from Buddhism by Buddha's follower Saraha in the same way that Zen was created by Bodidharma.

Saraha is the founder of Tantra; the vision to transform duality and set us free.

Saraha has a fascinating story. He was the son of a very learned Brahmin who had a very high rank in the court of the local king Mahapala. All his family was very distinguished, highly privileged scholars and Saraha was the youngest and the most intelligent of them all. The king loved him very much and wanted him to marry his daughter.

However, Saraha had other ideas, he wanted to renounce everything, he wanted to become a sannyasin. As you can imagine this created a little bit of controversy, the King was hurt as Saraha was a famous Brahmin, a handsome young fellow, so intelligent with such a great future waiting for him.

Saraha became a disciple to Sri Kirti who told him to forget all that he learned, all his vedas, and all your learning and all your nonsense. That it is perhaps the most difficult to unlearn, your intellectual capital is the most difficult to give up. And then how? How can we unlearn, how can we become ignorant again? To become innocent like a child is the greatest austerity.

Saraha became a great meditator and he managed to set your mind free. By now he became famous for being a great meditator and fresh and light like a new leaf. Then he had a vision. He saw a woman in the marketplace who would become his real teacher.

And that it is a sine qua non-characteristic of Tantra; it is a female energy. It is the few religions that is not misogynist nor chauvinistic male centred.

In fact, to go into Tantra one will need the cooperation of a wise woman; without her one would not be able to enter Tantra's complex world.

Saraha left his master and went to the market looking for this woman and he found her there. She was an arrow maker woman. She was there, so earthly, vibrant and vital, so rooted to the ground, visceral and ardent, so real, savage, unrefined, connected to Mother Earth, to creation and exuding freedom.

He immediately felt something extraordinary that he never felt before; in her presence, he felt something so fresh emanating from the source.

She was a woman of action and completely absorbed in her action.

He approached her and asked if she was a professional smith to what she laughed and said to him that he was a Brahmin who left his vedas, that now he was following Buddha's teachings and what was the point of changing books if he was still being the same stupid man! She was laughing so openly, so coarse and yet she was a magnet and he could not go away, he was an iron glued to that magnet.

Then she asked him; "Are you a Buddhist? Buddha's meaning can only can only be known through actions, not through words. Do not waste any more of your time and follow me".

For the first time, he understood the Buddha's teaching of being in the middle and to avoid any excess, any extreme. He was a philosopher then he became an anti-philosopher from one extreme to the other, worshiping one subject then worshiping the next but worshiping nevertheless.

The middle point is where transcendence happens. To be focused and absorbed in the middle is meditation and the wisdom that comes from it.

From meditation comes an action that triggers a change. We have to be in action, self- absorbed in it, so passionate and intensely submerged in it, to become one with it, to be total in action is to be free of action.

The legend says she was not really a woman she was a hidden buddha who came to help this man to find his greatest potential. Why a woman? Because Tantra believes that as a man has to be born from a woman so the new birth of a disciple has also to come out of a woman.

In fact, all the masters have a feminine energy, a grace a beauty a peaceful maternal energy that nourishes you for as long as you need. It does not matter if you have a male form, the energy is a maternal one, a creational one that gives birth to the new you. The master chooses the disciples, the master waits for them. He can penetrate all the possibilities and potential of their disciples. A disciple cannot choose a master as the disciple is blind and ignorant. If you start feelings for your master, it means that he is already in your heart transforming your energies.

Saraha found his soul mate, they were in such immense love, so submerged in each other. She taught him Tantra and he became a Tantrika under her supervision and guidance.

Once I went to a talk by a Guru from Mauritius who was visiting the UK. He was Swami Paramananda, a wonderful man. Someone, nervously again, asked him about Tantra.

He explained that Tantra was a force, an energy of action, where the opposites fuse so intensely that they become one. Where you can change, and transform and set yourself free as all become one and you achieved detachment from the source of pain.

As the object of attachment implies the fear of not having enough of it, and the need to go over and over again implies a separation from the object and yourself, through Tantra you take action and become one with the object therefore do not need to re-visit it again.

He gave an example. He asked to imagine that you want to quit smoking. Then you start smoking, so mindfully, so intensely, observing and feeling each time the cigarette is against your lips. You feel with the whole intensity, you are so focused that you stop existing. It is only the action of smoking, how it goes into your mouth, the taste, the feel, the smell, the flavour; like in a hyper stimulation of all the senses. You smoke it and feel it in your lungs, the exchange of air, the expiration. Then you smoke another and another until you satiate all desire, completely self-absorbed, all meaningful, all action, until it becomes nothing, until it is part of you, no separation, no need to crave it or desire it as it is no longer external to your own-self.

It becomes a memory that is part of your map and you do not need the cigarette to find it. Then you quit smoking, no need to do it again!

Imagine you are an archer. There, you are in the middle of a beautiful field; the sun is shining and the trees are dancing with the wind. A little tune is playing. The movement of the branches are in tune with a gentle breeze that caresses your face. The ground is in a deep green grass, holding your feet and giving you a perfect, solid stand.

You are there, staring at your goal fixed a hundred yards away from you. You can see it afar, a round circle, impenetrable solid hay painted in white with perfect black circumferences in an ascending count, 1, 2, 3,4... then after nine, nothing! Just the middle, the focus, the perfect circle. Your goal is the core, right in the centre the neutral one!

Then you grasp the bow, you feel it, you sense its strength, how tense is its cord; a hard and strong opponent that needs to be bound. You reach for the arrow; a straight, sleek, smooth and penetrating projectile converging in a point.

You tense the bow with the arrow at your eye level, and in that instant, you are one with the arrow. You become the arrow.

There is not field, or trees, no grass, no thoughts. You are not thinking of anything else, you are not thinking of how gravity has claimed your Mammary glands and other appendices. You are not thinking of your grey hairs; neither you are thinking of your past, your traumas, what your mother did to you or did not do! You are not thinking of paying bills, buying milk and eggs for breakfast next day. There are not thoughts about what would happen to you in 10 years' time, nor what are you having for dinner, neither are you thinking of sex! No, you are nothing of that sort, you are an arrow   !

Then you are aiming and the arrow is the extension of your consciousness that it is already in the target. You are aiming straight not to the 1, or 4 ring, neither to the left or to the right. Then, you are in the air flying with only one thing in view the target that it is closer and closer and closer. It is not a circle anymore, it is a bigger entity, it is not a round shape it is just an IT!

You hit it! You are in, you penetrate it, you fuse and become one with the aimed core. Your consciousness is in it! There is nothing else, you win it, you reach the zenith and become one with it. The orgasmic impact was fulfilled and the explosion of energy was released.

Then your mind goes silent, fulfilled and satisfied, the job is done! You got pleasure as you feel a liberation, an inner joy.

When your mind accomplishes its goals, it becomes quiet. The mind does not like unfinished businesses. If you had hit a 4 or even a 9, you would try again as you did not aim correctly. Your mind, starts making calculations, and thinking of so many other possibilities. It starts doubting of one's abilities to succeed. Then it may start thinking of how fat, old and ugly your body may be. That in the old good days you may hit the target or thinking of the milk and bread for the next day. It will blame the wind, or the light or the bow for your failure, as even a 9 is a failure.

We bring judgment and distress to the equation, our ego criticises us, put us down. We forget it is sunny and gorgeous out there. We bring anger, resentfulness and envy other archers who hit the jackpot! You created techniques, superstitions, request divine intervention, to hit the target. Those who hit it before you become "experts" and you admired them and think they are superior to you! They may help you to remember that you are the archer who became one with the bow, who then became one with the arrow, then the arrow that it is you united you with your target and you fuse with it and you become one. If you target is a 4 or a 6, or even the circle in the middle, a perfect 10, it does not matter, the trajectory is the same a straight line, no judgment, neutral position, no thought only you. Your target is not a circle anymore, it is a circle crossed by an arrow. It got transformed, fulfilled, achieved so it is not a target anymore.

When you accomplish it, you feel pleasure, you experience beauty, you feel joy and there are not thoughts anymore, just you with your inner joy and there is mind no more.

Your pleasure senses have satisfied all that they can feel, an ecstasy, a transformation, has been reached and that momentum stays with you.

That moment is silent, that ecstasy is wordless, an orgasmic language that is a separated entity from your mind. It communicates with reality and transforms it; it is real and has the power to liberate you.

The same happens to all attachments, including sex, to all sufferings, to all concepts. To become one, a unity and to transform.

To conclude my little introduction to Tantra I leave you with one of Saraha's principle:

The human reality is the only way to go to the ultimate reality. It is only through our own experiences, bodies, feelings, emotions as that it is what we are. We can just move on from the place where we are. Sex is a reality, and we can achieve Samadhi (it is a state of intense concentration achieved through meditation. In yoga, this is regarded as the final stage, at which union with the divine is reached, a blessing, a moment of ecstasy with the Divine) through it. The body is our reality, bodilessness can be reached through it. External is your reality; the inherent can be reached through it. All you need is to take action, no need to wait.

Love

What is love? What is your understanding of love? Where does it start and where does it finish? Is there more than one love? How do you feel love?

What is love? Is there a mental process that semantically describes LOVE? Perhaps love is all the rest, that we cannot describe with words. Perhaps it is that force, that indecipherable halo we can feel but we cannot own.

Perhaps it is that life force that compels us to be conscious of life itself.

Alternatively, it can be the Universe, the momentum, the force of expansion. It may be the whole consciousness that manifests our reality.

Yet, when I felt Drew growing inside of me, I found love so intense yet so intimate, so delicate, so fragile. When I look at my dog I genuinely feel love for him and from him.

I love being in meditation and I love God above any other love. I love myself as I am a manifestation of God's love. Is Love God itself? I do not know, However, whatever love may mean is beyond me as I do not need to know it, to describe it. I feel it and from that universal force all the good feelings and emotions emerge. Life itself comes from it and I love life and it compels me to be kind, giving, compassionate, helpful, selfless. It heals me and provides me the ability to forgive.

It makes me who I am and gives me a frame, a scaffolding of happiness. It brings joy and freedom and helps me to detach from hope and has brought me acceptance.

It gives me the force and the courage and the strength of a goddess. A lioness on the planes, with majesty, honour and pride.

I do not need to know what it is as it is nothing and everything.

Gratitude

According to the dictionary, gratitude is "Having the attitude of being Gratus (Latin word that means thankful, pleasing)"

When you are grateful, you are happy by what someone did for you and pleased by the results of their actions. It is the conclusion, the end of the story. A fact accompli!

Unlike indebtedness, you are not anxious about having to pay it back. By saying "Thank you", you are free.

Also, by saying "thank you" before the action is taken, it becomes powerful, as action has to take place as gratitude is already given. So, it has the power to set you free and also to command action to take place.

Think of an example, when you ask for something. Can I have the Ketchup, please. Thank you! Someone, somehow will pass it to you!

Another example is when you pray and show gratitude to God. "Thank you, God," for this or for that. The Divine formulae to receive gifts!

As we command our minds to manifest a determined reality as we have already close it and give the instruction to be accomplished.

Gratitude also makes you feel good, it sets you free from suffering.

It brings abundance and peace. It brings healing to your aching ill body when we are grateful to it.

We create a connection through Gratitude. We express love with gratitude.

We honour and respect through gratitude. Gratitude inspires noble feelings, compassion, consideration, empathy.

It releases us from fear and brings peacefulness when we confront our foes.

When we are grateful for any and everything in our life; good, bad and ugly, we set our mind free.

Sex

Sex is fun! Enjoy it!

However, I will tell you what is not sex. It is not a tool. It is not a currency, it is not a practice to satisfy your voyeurism. It is not porno nor an adult industry. It is not prostitution, neither is it an addiction, it is not a taboo, it is not masturbation. It is neither a tool of moral judgement. It is not a physical exercise or a series of repetitive sinuous movements and postures.

Sex is not dirty, neither clean, it is what it is, it is sex. It is not shameful, it is not evil. It is not promiscuous or even casual. It is not the cause of pain or disrepute. Sex is not violence nor a mechanism to slave one to another.

Sex is not procreation or marriage. Sex is not female neither male. Sex is only what it is. Your sexual orientation is irrelevant, sex is sex and nothing else. Sex makes us equal. Sex is not judgment, it does not know if you are fat, old or ugly. Sex is not black, white, red or yellow, neither bisexual, gay or straight. Sex is not a perfume or an aphrodisiac, also it is not seductive underwear on a hairless body.

Sex is sex and that it is what it is.

It is you and it is part of you. We love it and enjoy it, therefore we respect it, honour it and detach ourselves from it. As sex is an independent entity, a force that does not belong to us.

Sex is an energy, a force, a vehicle that transports us to Godly places. Sex is holy and powerful that brings joy and quietens the mind in the moment of ecstasy.

Sex is Tantra, it is strong, it is genuine, it is passion, it gives, it nourishes, it teaches us. Through sex we reach the power of creation. We create other beings that are born from us. Through it we express closeness, intimacy and love for each other.

Sex brings us the power to create ourselves, to sublimate that beautiful loving energy and become a better person, to excel in every field we wish. It reinvents us. It liberates us as it is the fusion of the separate being with the Universe. When you reach that connection, you need nothing, not even a sexual partner, nothing. You are one with that energy, with that passion and you can manifest it in every aspect of your life.

However, when we lose the meaning of sex, when we deal with an energy that we do not honour, respect or know how to handle it; we only bring suffering and unhappiness. We get lost and distort in our own reality. What is diaphanous and affectionate becomes evil, devious and murky.

Love yourself and love your sexuality. Make love in total fusion with your sex partner. Observe, feel, embrace, have orgasms and become one. Be mindful and honest. Act with integrity and detachment. Honour your bodies and love them.

It empowers you and makes your life joyful and fun! So, have mindful sex and be free!

Yoga is a Scientific Method

Yoga means the scientific method to reach oneness most likely developed around the sixth and fifth centuries BC. It is a series of techniques developed to unify mind and spirit. One of the processes through which you can achieve to quieten your mind and connect with the universal melody, a song of divine lyrics.

In the same way that Bodhidharma was concerned about the monks about their physical health while dealing with the rigorous discipline of meditation and created a series of physical exercises (that it became Kung Fu) Yoga has a physical element.

The Asanas (postures) are design to allow the energy to flow through the body. To strengthen the core, to stretch, to increase stamina, balance and overall to prepare the body for the mental and spiritual process during meditation.

We must think of our existence as a whole. Body, Mind and Spirit are part of who we are.

The ancient Greeks also considered that in order to have a healthy mind you should have a healthy body. According to Socrates, it was good to take exercise, to diet, take medication when needed, living within one's income.

Plato and Aristotle also follow the same current regarding a healthy living.

Then in the 1st century the Roman poet Juvenal in his Satire X wrote:

Mens sana in corpore sano (Latin phrase, usually translated as "a sound mind in a sound body")

He said we should pray to have a healthy mind in a healthy body... that was 20 centuries ago.

East and West for thousands of years have been concerned about the relationship between both; mind and body.

Yoga is more than taking a matt and putting your legs in the air, and force the body into acrobatics and showing off how flexible we are. It cannot be Yoga!

Yoga respects your own self as it brings wisdom and compassion. The first thing with Yoga is that there is no ego, it is not a competition. Yoga is love, so be gentle to yourself, do as much as you can, listen to your body and be compassionate and grateful to it, after all it is the only one you have. Be patient as time does not exist, your progress will be measured day by day. It is a progression, not a race.

Then we involve Ego and we create hundreds of modalities and my Yoga is better than yours. And mine is more complex, more difficult for you to do... More and more and more elements... more alien from its core, more western in order to satisfy the market.

Hot Yoga! What horror! Just because when you go to India and you practice Yoga in a tropical country and you sweat like a horse that now; wow, Eureka, we have to do Yoga in a super-hot room where we are going to aggress the body and push it, that our cardiovascular system will work harder, and we are going to get stronger...

Yoga is love, Yoga is spirituality and not aggression. Unfortunately, twisted versions of it became a business! When in fact, yoga is quiet, seeking simplicity to become nothingness.

Meditation

It is a method where you can reach a space above mental semantics. Where your mind is quiet and just being exposed to a contemplative state.

Meditation evolves, it is a practice where your brain learns to be disciplined. It gets the freedom to switch off and to create new neuropathic connections. An opportunity to expand your mind, to bring order and silence.

Meditation is also a bridge between your consciousness and a subconscious mind. It brings you an opportunity to reach higher levels of awareness and wisdom.

You can take ownership of your own mental process and learn how to meditate in the way that works for you. However, it is a practice, that you have to persevere. By giving up as you cannot put your mind in silence the first time you do it, is giving up prematurely. A baby learns to run after she learns to crawl and then to stand and then to walk.

Think of meditation as the chance to do a spring cleaning! Then, imagine yourself having a new mind, fresh, expanded, full of vitality and joy. It is like when you reboot your computer, and upload new updates. You can defragment the hard disk and create more space! Within this context, every little helps! If you just manage to clean 0.00000000000000001% of the hard disk at least you create a new space, that you did not have before.

Imagine you are on a holiday and you are in a pool alone, no one else making ripples, noises or disturbing the waters, and you are there floating in the middle, drifting, feeling totally relaxed and safe. It is a pool, you know where the edges are and nothing in it that may imply a danger. How does that make you feel? You just close your eyes and feel the movement of the water. You do not even feel your own body, there is not weight nor movement you just go with the flow!

At the beginning use your imagination to distract your mind. Start like a baby rolling over her body then discovering the coordinated action between bending the knees and straighten her arms! This is a guided meditation where you can have lots of fun and visualizing fantasies that will create pockets of crawls, moving forward in your process of mental clarification.

Some people get upset as they cannot visualize, they cannot imagine or follow what the guide is telling you to do and that it is okay too. We have different ways of perception, some are visual, others auditory and others we just know. Just listen and if images do not come to mind it is okay. If your shopping lists come across instead, it is okay too.

One of the simplest ways to meditate is to be aware of your own breathing, no forced, no deep, just simply ask your mind/brain to be attentive to your breathing, to observe your own breathing and nothing else.

Then, you can go towards a silent meditation, a journey inwards, travelling deeper and deeper, and deeper indeed. It is like drifting, floating in the ocean; where you are not in the pool anymore but it feels the same.

Nutrition and healthy lifestyle

We have seen so far why you deserve to be healthier, happier and free from suffering and pain. All because you are a miracle. You are beautiful, you are a complex organism in an evolutionary scale. You have a brain that communicates with a mind, that is in connection to a soul. You are unique, you are a vibrational intelligent energy that vibrates in different frequencies, manifested as matter in a conscious reality.

You are the guardian of the species, in your genes you bank the treasure of life.

You are love, you are sex, you are Tantra you are anything and everything you can dream of. You are art in movement, you are science, matter and energy. You are emotions, intelligence, knowledge and wisdom.

You are a smile, a kiss and a tender hug. You are an atom, you are a galaxy and even more.

As you are all that and more, how are you feeding yourself? What are you doing to look after the custodial flux of your existence?

I hope that by now you are starting to grasp how important you are. Your body deserves the best you can provide. Your body deserves your respect, your love and consideration. It is your temple, it is what makes you real, it gives you shape, it gives you opportunities of creation.

How could you exist in this realm if you did not have a body? A ghost? A memory from the past?

We are integrated beings where chemistry and physics mix to nourish our beautiful bodies.

For us to be in our prime condition, we require macro and micro nutrients, vitamins, minerals and water.

We require gases among them, oxygen to create a combustion and generate energy.

We require the mechanical actions and physical functions to transport, and distribute resources around the body. We also need to collect waste and detritus that our chemistry and metabolic functions have created to excrete them.

We are an ecosystem, a kingdom, where thousands of functions are working in unison, in a perfect melody that encompasses life.

All our functions are related, all of them are partners in the same enterprise. Everything depends on the same source of nourishment. All our organs are our workers, our arteries and veins are our motorways and roads. Our liver is our main industrialised source of resources.

Our respiratory system, the bridge to life. Arteries and veins connected to the heart, bring in and out precious cargo that connects us to the abstract world of volatile substances.

Our kidneys are the purification plant of residual waters. Our heart is the turbine that generates the energy, like a generator of the electrical system that illuminates in the middle of the night our roads and houses.

Our immune system is our police force and army. Fighting external invaders and keeping the house in order.

Our nervous system is the communicator, the coordinator. This system is our networking, our broadband; the postman, the commentator, the executioner and the decision maker.

We have our scaffolding, our statues of colossus holding us like Atlas supporting an inner world; benevolent bones and fearless muscles, powerful Adonis, workers of movement.

Our skin is our walls, our first line of defense; our borders and our definition, conscientious germinating layers that shed its bricks every 6 weeks. It is our boundaries, our organ of touch, our sovereign state with its ambassadors and diplomats.

Our endocrine system is our regulator. Councils that will determine our growth, our genre, our ability to reproduce, to rest, to attack, to make love, to care. They will nurse us and tell us when we stop being children and become adults. Teachers of lessons who anticipate our reactions and interactions.

Then our procreative system, the bank of our DNA ready to merge. It is our entrepreneurial asset, the articulate trampoline to immortality.

Our graceful lymphatic system; the sewage, the canal, the transporter. It does not only keep us from dirtiness but also works as barges navigating on milky waters transporting precious fats.

And then, we have the digestive one! How emblematic, what a powerful architect. The artist of them all. The semi-god, the provider.

Colonies of farmers in his entrails are generating nutrients to be shared. Selfless being that works for all.

Then it is you! What are the prime materials that are you putting in your mouth to feed all that majestic city? You are the one in charge! All of them depend on you!

I can spend hours and hours explaining to you all the metabolic functions, chemical reactions, production of enzymes, catalytic functions, physiology of each organ. Would you listen to me? Oh, silly ignorance that is killing you! A crime is committed with each bite!

Would you not be bored at the second I start talking about it, or defensive? Or would you give excuses, or take into consideration the emotional factors involved in the relationship between food and psyche. Would you be in denial and admit to eating half of the things you really eat if we analysed your eating behaviour? Would you avoid responsibility, blaming society, the media, the supermarkets, the buy 2 and get one free?

Are you praying for a new sugar substitute, and fat free products full of starch and other sugars in order to eat another piece of cake? Are you drinking diet Colas, as they are diet so who cares how many chemicals that my body cannot digest are in it?

People come to me, asking for help, they want to lose weight, they want to feel healthier. They do not understand why they are bloated, they have acne in the skin, cannot sleep, are gaining weight, their hormones are all over different places.

Then I ask to provide a full detailed food diary for a whole week, including the drinks, the quantities, the times of meals, if they were homemade cooked or ready meals.

They do not do it. They find it is too much to ask. It is so boring, time consuming and for those who do it, they are half way done. They forget over a third what they eat or drink and the record of alcoholic consumption goes to the stupor of the hypnotic allure of Morpheus' kingdom.

So, what are you eating? What are you drinking and how much? How much exercise do you do? Do you know what exercise does for your body? Are you not at least curious?

In sum, I recommend you to have an alkalizing diet. An alkalasing diet will neutralise the reaction of excess acidity in your body. Your inner kingdom requires a homeostatic environment and a balanced pH. The body has the tendency to have an alkaline pH.

To give you an example: The normal blood pH is between 7.35 and 7.45.

A pH of 7 is neutral. Below pH 7 is acidic. A variety of factors affect blood pH including what is ingested, vomiting, diarrhea, lung function, endocrine function, kidney function, and urinary tract infections.

Your body is healthier when it is in its natural environment, the more acidic the more contaminated it is and that will trigger toxicity and disease.

CO_2 is acidic and excreted through exhalation by the lungs. Carbonated water, or bubbles in soda or water is CO_2. Why would someone drink something that the body has tried so hard to get rid of?

Also, drinking water in bottle. I know a lot is said about the plastic containers and the release of carcinogenic substances if temperature of the bottle is high, but please do check the pH in the label. What is the point in buying an acidic water?

General speaking vegetables and fruits are alkalising; lemon being one of the best. Then animal products are more acidic. Animal protein is a complex one. To break it down to amino acids it has to pass through several chemical reactions that produce byproducts and waste that are acidic. Sugar and processed food are acidic too.

Obesity makes the body acidic, also smoking and consumption of alcohol. Acidity taxes the body with a heavy duty. The body has to react and sacrifice a lot of their nutrients, anti-oxidants, minerals to neutralise the acid.

Liberation of free radicals that are like hand grenades, anti-personal mines, explosives that the body has to pay to be neutralised reduces the budget for other preventative services.

Also, the animal fibre that is not digested in the low intestine pass to the colon where starts a process of putrefaction and adheres to the intestinal wall. It creates an acidic environment reducing levels of Oxygen and increasing the proliferation of anaerobic microorganisms rising the toxicity in the body.

There are many more reasons why you should avoid animal products in general, mainly dairy, as an adult you do not require it and it may affect your immune and endocrine system due to the levels of hormones and antibodies. Also with the industrialised production of milk, where cows are constantly lactating and confined to small compacted spaces are injected with lots of antibiotics and hormones that you will drink.

When people suggest to you to reduce consumption of animal products and perhaps to become vegetarian please listen. Not only is it good for your health but plenty of cows, chicks, lambs and horses will be grateful!

Then, how much water do you drink?

Water, life force in liquid form!

Much of the universe's water is created as a byproduct of star formation.

Perhaps water is present in other worlds, after all, its components, hydrogen and oxygen, are among the most abundant elements in the universe.

On Earth, water is covering 71% of its surface.

Water's properties are critical for the proliferation of life as it allows replication. All known forms of life depend on water. Water is vital both as a solvent in which many of the body's solutes dissolve and as an essential part of many metabolic processes within the body.

One of the essential uses of water is during the process of Metabolism. This is the process where we can break down molecules to assimilate its elements or create bigger structures, larger molecules for different functions in the body.

Metabolism is divided into Anabolism and Catabolism. In Anabolism, water is removed from molecules (through enzymatic chemical reactions) to grow larger molecules (e.g. starches, triglycerides and proteins for storage of fuels and information).

In Catabolism, water is used to break bonds to generate smaller molecules (e.g. glucose, fatty acids and amino acids to be used for fuels for energy use or other purposes). Without water, these metabolic processes could not exist.

Water is fundamental to photosynthesis and respiration. The photosynthetic cells in plants use the sun's energy to separate hydrogen from oxygen in water. Hydrogen is combined with CO_2 (absorbed from air or water) to form glucose and oxygen is released.

In the cellular respiration (ours), we take the oxygen produced by the plants and use it as fuel. From that operation, we exhale water and CO_2.

Water is also central to acid-base neutrality and enzyme function. Water is considered in its natural form to be neutral, therefore pH 7 (pH can be altered by the addition of natural salts and other minerals).

The human body contains from 55% to 76% water, depending on body size. To function properly, the body requires between one and seven litres of water per day to avoid dehydration.

The precise amount depends on the level of activity, temperature, humidity, genre, size and other factors.

Most of the water we require is ingested through foods (20%) or drinks including drinking water.

Consensus agrees that approximately 2 liters (6 to 7 glasses) of water daily is the minimum to maintain proper hydration.

Men should consume 3.0 liters and women 2.2 liters; pregnant women and breastfeeding women should increase their intake.

Please be advised, that despite its liquid form, alcohol does not count!

Also, some authors consider coffee and tea dehydrate so they should not count either.

The body is noble and graceful, it is a loyal companion that will sacrifice itself to follow you.

Our emotions also, affect our body. The messenger can store them in different areas. The Stress councils will allocate the tariff in energy units. Again, the poor body has to pay the price.

We constantly submit our bodies to stress, pollution, fatigue, lack of sleep, poor diets, bad posture, chemicals on cosmetics, clothing, cleaning products and any other place you may fancy.

We change the colour of our hair, we use hair remover, nail polish and their remover. We bleach the smile, we stifle with heat our poor hair. We drink in excess, we eat healthy food in scarcity as the race against time has reached our fields where they plant, plant, plant, with no permission for the land to rest.

We are connected to phones, IPod, tablets, laptops and when we are at work we are also on the phone, on the desktop and so, and so. We are under constant bombardment from marketing campaigns, buy, buy, buy... buy even if you do not have the money... Carry on buying money to buy, buy, buy...

Buy food, and more food, rubbish food, food that is fast food as you need more time to buy and get fat and buy, and buy, and buy slimming pills to make your body suffer even more...

And if you are on the other side of the coin; sell, sell, sell and carry on selling if you want to be paid, paid, paid and get money to buy, buy, buy.

We are so busy, it is a sitting down marathon out there. No time to stop, to rest, to contemplate, to say to the body: I am listening to you; I want to say thank you, I am so grateful to you my dearest friend, my sweet companion.

It seems there is no time to say sorry, I am demanding so much of you or even a simply I love you my dear body.

Body needs rest, it needs to sleep, to slow down and have periods of solitude and silence.

Your body needs to relax in order to mend and heal itself. We need at least 8 hours per day of sleep to carry out all the metabolic functions and repairs we need to keep the body youthful and healthy.

The body needs to slow down and relax, perhaps try a good massage that will not only help you to relax but it will stimulate all the bodily functions to reach homeostasis.

Our body is alive, and it is a dynamic being that it is constantly interacting between its inner self and the external world. The body needs movement, it needs exercise (thought, it does not need to be put under too much exerting exercise that it may cause further injuries).

To give you just one example; our body has designed fantastic hydraulic systems to save energy and make it even more efficient.

We know arterial blood is propelled by the rhythmic beat of the heart. Venous blood that travels against gravity towards the heart and its comrade, the loyal companion, lymph gets their push by their eyeful friends, the muscles. When these contract, they generate a force that squeezes, in an exquisite tempo, our bodily fluids like gilded currents transiting through the locks of a canal.

PART 3

I.S Healing System™

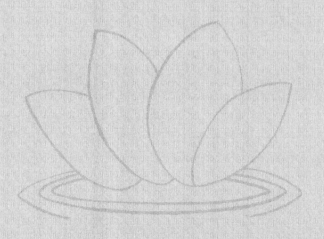

I.S Healing System™

Not to be confused with I.S, so called Islamic State.

I decided to reclaim the letters I and S. We cannot allow the semantics of a terrorist organization to claim ownership of I.S.

"Is" is the present form of the Verb BE. It denotes existence! We cannot allow a group of individuals who wants to annihilate to have ownership of Existence!

"Is" is also the plural of the Greek letter "Iota".

Iota *noun*

1. the ninth letter of the Greek alphabet (Ι, ι), transliterated as 'i'

2. an extremely small amount. A smidgen speck that sometimes we ignore or we consider unimportant.

    "nothing she said seemed to make an iota of difference"

1. Meaning of 9 in numerology:

From a purely mathematical perspective, the number 9 is sui generis.

When you multiply any number by 9, then add the resulting digits and reduce them to a single digit, it always becomes a 9. For example, 5 x 9 = 45, reduce 45 to a single digit by adding them together: 4 + 5 = 9. Similarly, 9 x 9 = 81, and 8 + 1 = 9. Or 25 x 9 = 225, 2 + 2 + 5 = 9, 3456 x 9 = 31,104 = 3+1+1+0+4 = 9, and so on.

Any number multiplied by 9 reduces to 9.

Any number that was multiplied by 9 takes on the characteristics of the 9.

No other number holds that quality.

The 9 is also the last of the cardinal numbers. You can associate this as the last resource, the ultimate goal, the end of a series of events.

Number 9 is the number of Universal love, belief, enlightenment, spiritual awareness and expansion, wisdom, positivism, helpfulness, generosity, drive, inner-strength, management, responsibility, intuition, strength of character and natural leadership.

The number 9 reverberates with the ability to say 'No'. It is important to validate and recognize our boundaries and say NO.

Other characteristics of 9 are:

Integrity, honesty, creativity, loyalty, resourcefulness, wisdom, self-esteem, freedom, charisma, tolerance, humility, altruism, sensitivity, and benevolence.

Also, empathy, open mindedness, communication skillfulness, understanding, forgiveness, compassion, gratitude.

The 9 is a symbol that offers warmth and compassion to everyone; unconditional love to the world; it has a global consciousness.

The 9 understands humankind. The 9 is non-judgmental, it is kind and tolerant and it is the most mindful of numbers.

The qualities of the number 9 are those of leadership, the ability to see clearly, integration of the physical, intellectual, spiritual.

It understands unity, truth, concord and dissolves attachments.

And that is why I want you to associate the I, as the individual, the person to absorb the characteristics of the number 9, as I (Iota) is the ninth letter of the Greek alphabet.

You are the "I" as the entity, the person who deserves to witness the characteristics of the number 9 manifested in your life.

My desire is for you to create a thought, a mental pattern that at any time that you have doubt, you have pain, you are confused you associate your -self with the properties of the number 9. We scientifically, mathematically proved that any figure factorized by 9 is equal to nine when we add their individual ciphers. Your mind is accepting this as a valid fact as you have tried and proved it.

Imagine that you are swimming in the deep ocean and you are tired and it is getting dark and you do not know how far you are from shore, you are afraid as you start imagining sharks coming for you underneath from the abyss, from the unknown. You can see them, you can feel them tearing you apart.

Suddenly a buoy, there, right in front of you, not any time soon, as the water is getting agitated, the cadence of the waves is seesawing aggressively. At that point, it starts raining so heavily, each drop is like needles perforating all your senses; the roar of the wind is leaving you earless and then, there is this beacon, full of light, full of hope in the shape of 9.

What do you do? What do... YOU... DO? YOU GRAB IT, you grab it with all your strength as if there were no tomorrow, as your life depends on it. You close your eyes and you become that beacon, that 9.

It does not matter if you believe in numerology or in Universal Laws or in Spirituality, you just inform your mind and force your brain to create patterns of association that nine, that Iota (i), are the symbol of what you admire and bring you peace.

1.a. Iota transliterates as "I" or "i", therefore you can read it also as the subject pronoun "I".

In grammar, there are three types of pronouns: subject (for example, they); object (him, her them); or possessive (your, their).

Therefore, we can associate Iota and its graphic form (I) as the pronoun I, like I am, I feel, I can... "I" can take ownership of Iota, I can identify with Iota, as already they have the same graphical representation.

This is another play of words for your brain to make connections to identify with what you want to integrate into your process of understanding.

We already know that our process of learning undergoes different steps. From pure subconscious ignorance to subconscious knowledge, where we act automatically, we do not know how we get the information we only know we can act upon it.

The more connections, the more patterns we create; and then the more autonomous the learning process becomes.

2. An extremely small amount.

From Macro to Micro. How to decompose a whole structure to its minimum components, their most miniscule imprint in order to understand, to release and to overcome any issue.

When I was a student I had a teacher, who asked us to learn and remember by heart all the Anatomy Compendium. We were terrified at the prospect but she reassured us by using the analogy "you can eat the whole elephant by cutting it into little pieces".

What are your elephants? How complex are they? How old are they? And how to start "eating" and digest them to excrete them.

How to go so deep, to the extremely small that it will disappear and stop causing harm.

We have the perception that bigger is better. We get impressed and sometimes intimidated by ostentatious, dramatic events or by those who have more money, bigger cars, bigger houses, bigger muscles... (you get the picture).

Remember Iota means 'something that it is small that it is insignificant'.

Again, bringing judgement based on the ego. We have the tendency to value what it is big, difficult, expensive, with an apparent power. We get intimidated and value their labels, their names, their locations. We pay for being associated with their names.

Many years ago, I had a client who had a terrible pain on his left side, by his pancreas. He had been everywhere as no one could "find anything". He was desperate as his last resource was going to Harley Street and after he spent thousands of pounds, in every imaginable test, they said that the results indicated he had nothing.

How could it be possible for him to dare to feel pain after Harley Street said he had nothing. He came to me with no hope, skeptical about me. What could I do to take his pain away after all I was miles away from Harley Street. He did not believe either in any of my therapies and Reiki and energy work was charlatanism.

He constantly was saying to me, in Harley Street they did this test, they put me in X machine, an eminent doctor saw me and so on and so on. It was an excellent practice right in the middle of Harley Street.

I treated him for a few hours, he gave me if I remembered well around £60.

He was pain free. And he never came back. He thought it was by chance he released his pain, after all, it might be nothing as Harley Street told him so.

I do not have anything against the practitioners (they may be very good professionals), who work in that road or of the prices they charge for their services. I am neither against those desperately finding locations alongside Harley Street to be caught in its reputation. I just find it curious that it became a question of snobbish status.

The gentleman I mentioned was not the only one coming to me and saying " I have been in Harley Street!" As if by a miracle, the virtue of the name of a stretch of a road surrounded by bricks and mortar would heal you.

We forgot that the insignificant is significant. What is simple is complex in its own right.

Humble, innocent, transparent, inexpensive, easy are beautiful sincere attributes. Seek to be genuine and with essential qualities of honesty and integrity. Do not be afraid of being simple and free.

We have the tendency to undervalue them as if we were still at the times of the caverns; where we mate with the strongest of the tribesmen to bring up a strong offspring. It seems we have not evolved from the need to impress and disempower others for us to feel we are in an elite.

We have the need to have status, therefore we need labels. Labels are the easiest way to send that message. They are visual symbols saying you cannot afford what I have. You do not belong to my class. It differentiates us from others. One may argue they are beautifully designed, they have high quality, a reputation of craftsmanship and savoir faire that justify their prices.

Also, they represent an image, a conveyed message crafted by ingenious and cunning advertising companies. A message that it is part of your personality.

To give you an example, what makes a man wear a belt in his trousers? You may say it may be for two reasons; one is practical, to hold them in place and avoid them going down, as an antigravity tool and/or a fashion accessory; as with skinny jeans they would hardly fall down by themselves.

Now, does the belt needs a buckle, yes of course as it needs to lock the belt. Does this buckle need to be big and ostentatious? No need as a buckle is a buckle and size and shape will not alter its function. Does this buckle require to be a Louis Vuitton? What is the need to have a big L and V on top of the groin? Only the owner can reply to that one!

We have the tendency to discard what it is simple, clear, small, essential. We do not see it. We do not look at the obvious. When we are so overwhelmed by events we do not think in organelles or cells or going deeper in the cloud of electrons or quantum particles jumping and manifesting energy while being observed.

We could not function if that was the case, as at microscopic level we are also a macro Universe. However, as human beings, we are also a speckle in the planet, and the planet is a speckle in the universe.

Everything is relative but all is connected. The interaction of our electrons' clouds is connected with the universe according to the laws of thermodynamics.

One of the laws that catches my attention and allow us to be philosophical, is the second Law of thermodynamics.

It speaks of a beautiful concept. ENTROPY.

Entropy is a measure of disorder, chaos that, in a closed environment, it can only increase. Being messy, barbaric is natural and the closer the surroundings are, the bigger they will grow.

What "disorder" refers to is the number of different minuscule states a system can be in, a random proportion that we cannot determine. By "microscopic states", we mean the exact states of all the fragments making up the system.

The idea here is that just knowing the bigger aspects in a composition, does not tell us much about the exact state of each particle making up the system. For even a very small piece of matter, there can be trillions of different microscopic states, all of which correspond to the composition.

A way to think of the second law of thermodynamics is to imagine your mind; a mind, if not cleaned and tidied, will invariably become more messy and disorderly with time - regardless of how attentive one is at keeping it clear. When the mind is cleaned, its entropy decreases.

The more closed our mind is, the higher the entropy is and by expanding the container the entropy will dissipate.

In summary, to clarify the big picture we have not only to be aware of the iota but to understand its role and how it can trigger a change with repercussions not only in you as individual but, in the manner you interact with others and your community.

Now, do you want to learn a method to reduce the mental entropy? I will tell you how.

The first ingredient you need is LOVE. Love yourself. Love and emotions are powerful energies. Love is the impetus, that triggers the motivation (Force) for you to act.

"I LOVE myself" is a powerful statement. It is the absolute harmony and balancer in the equation.

I LOVE myself then I can accept myself just in the way I am.

We already know that there is a portion of us that is in constant disorder, we are 100% perfect in the way we are, in fact by having disorder and chaos we embrace all that exists. We need all sort of opposites to be whole.

We are a micro universe part of a whole universe and we have all the properties of the micro and the macro.

We are a manifestation of love in a determined state of consciousness.

We now understand that we obey universal laws that we belong to the reality of energy in constant flux.

Nothing in us is superfluous or futile, we are wonderful just in the way we are thus One loves oneself.

Through love and compassion, we create a conscious understanding of our reality.

Through understanding we can achieve wisdom and knowledge of our Iotas; our own I.S Healing System™.

I to Identify

O to Observe

T to Transform

A to Accomplish

S to Set Free /Self-Realization

Now you know what "I.S" Healing System™ is; how are we going to approach it?

So far, we have seen the role of semantics. How our brain dialogues with the concept of a conscious mind. We have seen how important are words and how they trigger creation of thoughts that become a truth. Then, they manifest as a reality. We create neuropathic connections and it becomes a repetitive neurological action cementing its connections, making it even more difficult to dismantle and eradicate them from the system.

It is like creating motorways where we reroute the traffic from other directions, making them obsolete. The "public" will protest against the change as how is it possible that a perfect route that costs a lot of effort to be built can now become a white elephant! "That route had a destination, a perfectly rational destination that brought us an outcome, now are you coming to tell me that all that was for nothing" the brains says.

In Physics, we have another interesting law. The Law of Inertia.

Classic Physics established that we have the tendency to be inert. Not to change as change involves the input of a force, therefore the use of energy.

Since Aristotle then to Galileo and then Newton in his First Law of Motion; he describes inertia as an object not subject to any net external force moves at a constant velocity. Therefore, an object will continue moving at its current velocity until some force causes its speed or direction to change.

As we can see, it is perfectly understandable that our brain protests against change, after all, we are a physical, natural phenomenon.

Do we have to create a force to trigger a change? Change that subsequently will confront the laws of cause and effect and the law of conservation of energy.

So, where to start, we already know that by nature we have the tendency to carry on as usual, if we tried to change our change will trigger a reaction and our universe has the tendency to conserve energy. Change is not created our energy is constant we just can transform it.

That is the essence, transformation, as we cannot create we just transform it. We are going to transform our motorways!

Rene Descartes, French philosopher, scientist and mathematician who lived in the XVII century, and, considered the father of modern philosophy, stated: "I think, therefore I am", Thought then existence.

In his Discourse on the Method of Rightly Conducting the Reason and Seeking Truth in the Sciences, published in 1637, he wrote: ... resolving to seek no knowledge other than that of which could be found in myself or else in the great book of the world.

Descartes believed in emptying all preconceived and inherited notions, and starting fresh, putting back one by one the things that were undoubtfully truth, which for him started with the validation "I exist".

From Descartes, we can deduce several things. One of them is that existence as a conscious reality is based on thought. Thought that is conceived in the mind.

The mind creates a dialogue, a picture, an image, a sound. It produces a mental concept that triggers a neuropathic connection. I think therefore I am.

However, we can overthink, we can create far too many dialogues, idle talking, gossiping. Going around and around creating pseudo-existences that cannot be manifested at once creating havoc and mayhem therefore Anxiety.

How many times we do not hear from people saying that they are avoiding being in the company of other people as they cannot stop making negative assumptions, gossiping and putting people down. People talking and talking and talking like a mental diarrhea.

So, can you realise you are doing the same thing with your own inner dialogue? Are you avoiding the old ravenous discourse which will pull you out of your mind?

By overthinking you are not existing even more!

From Descartes and the current of Rationalism we get that the source of knowledge or justification comes from an intellectual and deductive reason. The truth excludes any empiric or sensorial experiences, beliefs, emotions, etc.

This current is still influencing our thinking today. This is the reason why we think science and its demonstrations and mathematical and scientific methodology and proof is more valid than other mental avenues.

Napoleon lost the Battle of Trafalgar but it seems the French ended conquering our thinking!

Rationalism is opposed to sensory experience or any religious teachings as a source of truth.

Again, our minds play around putting things in little folders separating intellectual reasoning from emotions. We validate and discard assumptions just because they belong to a folder or another; without realising we are the sum of the whole parts.

We lose balance and equilibrium when we try to credit one over another. We cannot suppress our emotions, or beliefs nor ignore our own bodies. Neither can we avoid intellectual reasoning and its acumen.

Lucky for us, after Descartes and the XVIII century's Enlightment, we got Kierkegaard, an absolute wonderful man, who was the pillar for Existentialism.

He believed that each one of us lives as a unique individual; giving priority to concrete human reality and emphasizing the importance of personal choice and commitment.

Existentialism is based on belief that philosophical thinking begins with the human being as a whole and not merely the thinking subject, but the acting, feeling, the living being. The strongest values of the existentialist thought are freedom and authenticity.

So far, we have seen here that we are everything, matter, biology, physics, religion, emotions, body, we are contradiction, order and chaos, and so and so, we are everything and nothing!

Why should we limit our perception of knowledge with bias egocentric preponderant concepts?

Body, mind, emotions, spirit, energy work together like different musical instruments playing the symphony of life!

Are you ready to approach your I.S now? Okay, here we go together!

We have learnt that new things by nature scare us and change is difficult. Also, that making an effort is taxing and we are prone to go with what we ae familiar, and we need a big input and consistency in order to make patterns change.

We also understood, why we have to be convinced in a rational, scientific manner in order to believe in a process.

We could see that we are complex, several things can affect us in a given situation, and they can trigger a series of reactions; our body reacts, our emotions and mental thoughts also react. Everything has a cause and an effect.

We have seen a lot of different concepts and studied ideas from other people who have molded our collective and cultural thinking.

We learnt that our mind can hurt us more than what comes from "outside". Inner dialogue can be idle and self -destructive. Also, we realise that we have a natural process of learning from totally unconscious ignorance to consciously ignorant, to consciously knowledgeable to unconsciously knowledgeable when things came as a second nature.

I have created for you this system in an organically way. It will become a second nature that we can learn by association.

I want to do an analogy comparing IS to the digestive system. There is nothing more basic and intrinsic to us than the need to nourish and survive.

I to Identify

We identify food. We recognised it through our senses. Our eyes, nose, hands, then our mouth are all involved in the process of identification. See an apple tree. You can visually identify the fruit, you pick up the apple and you smell it, you touch it. You can assess its consistency, its size, colour, texture. All this information will tell you that it is right to bring it to your mouth. Then you take an action to bite and bring it into your body.

O to Observe

In the mouth an observation takes place. Your teeth determine the material, how hard is and the resistance in order to break it down. Chemical reactions occur. You produce Saliva, that enrobes the macerated crumble memory of the apple. Your tongue observes the interaction of the juices and segment like a dance that at each turn is revealing more secrets.

It can detect the sweetness, the bitterness, the sour, or the absence of salt in the apple. The sweet sugars start breaking down giving away their chains or carbohydrates. Energy is leaking and your mouth is observing how the pieces disappear and become part of your body then it swallows.

The stomach receives the memory of apple via a toboggan of silky smoothness, your esophagus. Saliva has already informed him about the presence of food and he started to fill it with acid to dissolve and to Observe the gift it receives in an even deeper detail. Making things smaller and select what it is what. All that it is biologically toxic will peril in the acid. He goes around and around like a washing machine making things even smaller and observing and feeling what is what. Protein triggers a release of enzymes, breaking down chains of amino-acids, little bricks needed for further construction works.

T to Transform

Then, the stomach opens his gates, hermetic valves, so tightly firmly closed and pours his acidic content into the intestine.

Liver and Pancreas release transformative essences, to tame the corrosive acid and its contents. Transformation takes place as food as it was known is no more.

Then it travels hours and hours, long beautiful process, across metres and metres of tunnels, transforming the old distant reminiscence of apple and the process of absorption began.

A to Accomplish

Accomplishment of the process of absorption has taken place. We have extracted, squeezed until the last elixir of goodness. We finally understood what it is left behind has to go. We pass the baton on and open the gates. The ileocecal opens for a trip of non-return.

S to Set Free /Self-Realization

We have a last chance to reabsorb the little drops of goodness, the water of life. We go into the darkness aiming to release what does not work for us anymore. Toxic waste mixed with bulky fibre, provides a new atmosphere, new beings feeding from the gloom. But it does not matter as you know it has its reasons to exist. They are as valid as anything else and soon they are out of your system.

Peristalsis came at hand, a source of energy, a dynamic movement towards the gates of freedom. A release, an excretion has taken place. You can evacuate and set yourself free and you feel grateful!

Next time you go to the loo say thank you, please!

You have realised you have absorbed all the good and released what can stops you in your process of Enlightment.

Now that is the processes of our body. It requires energy to do so.

We have seen that according to the laws of Physics, we have the tendency to be inert. To keep the status quo. How can we trigger a process where we need energy to cause a reaction? Through our emotions. Emotions are energy.

One of the most powerful forces are intention and motivation. They are like the digestives juices that will neutralise your acidity and transform into nourishment all that soup of thoughts.

Act with honesty and a sincere genuine heart. And step by step. Take one episode at each time. Deconstruct it. How many emotions can you identify? Emotions are energies stored in different areas of the body. Feel where they are, go through the process to identify as you did for the apple.

I recommend you to choose a relaxing and peaceful place to reflect upon your Iotas. You can connect by remembering its meaning. Think of number nine and what it represents, also in Iota, and its meaning as the smallest thing. You are preparing yourself to go to an internal trip, you aim to reach the smallest, deepest of your shy hidden secrets and trigger a change and a release.

Start by a deep breathing. Slowly and rhythmic. Breath in, pause, breath out, pause. Do a few times this technique. It will trigger relaxation and a reduction of stress thanks to the stimulation of the Vagus nerve.

Close your eyes, and breath normally. Just have the intention to go deeper, and deeper and deeper into yourself.

At every step, reassure yourself that you are fine and you are safe and protected. You are just exploring and making an effort to know your best friend.

Then think of an event, or problem, emotion you may feel. Identify it, and break it down into little pieces, just by saying I am going deeper and deeper into myself. Scan your body, ask where in the body you are feeling the emotion, the energy or the disturbance. Do not think just feel it. Allow yourself to put your hands in the area you feel attracted to. Hold it, connect, and go deeper into it like a witness, an observer, then talk to your emotion. Tell her she has the right to manifest and has a voice to express the source of her pain.

Engage, think you are with a loved friend who is opening up and you feel lots of empathy and compassion. You listen but you do not judge. Then just allow things to be free and to take place. Show your gratitude, be grateful to your body who has been holding these energies in a safe place patiently waiting for you to take care of it.

Love your body and apologise for any abuse, mistreatment you have cause. Be grateful to the emotional energy who took a shape and a distinctive vibration for you to learn a lesson.

Emotion is an energy that flows, the nature is being in movement in constant flow, stagnant emotions are those that we have not dealt with and that have become our hostages. They willingly came to interact with us, partners in our quest of self-realisation. A quest of understanding and acceptance of expansion of our minds and their semantics. They got trapped in their efforts of helping us.

Stagnate waters running bitter, putrid and murky nesting obnoxious shady creatures that will poison your diaphanous nature.

Pain, disease and suffering grows from these springs of wretchedness. Fear becomes the banks of these uncirculated waters. The abyss of their depth is dark and scary, polluted with anger and violence. Ego and selfishness arise, lack of self-esteem and empathy governs. Pain and more pain, darkness, disbelief, cynicism and confusion await the sunset. We lose ourselves, we lose our power to see further into the horizon. We blame others, we blame the Gods, we blame the world and it is never our fault.

Breath and breath and carry on in your brave quest to reconnect with yourself. See your own self as a ray of sunshine, a provider of love, compassion and freedom. Open up the gates, allow the light to circulate. Transform the stagnant pond into a river and see it going to the sea of consciousness where each drop is water and each drop is a potential sea.

To end the exercise, you can breathe deeply again. Accept whatever emotion came across, even if you feel sad or in pain, or you may be crying, all that it is okay.

Bring your consciousness to your present moment, be aware of your toes, your feet, your legs, hips, chest, arms, hands, neck, head and face. Move them and feel you are completely grounded and awake.

Feel gratitude, feel emotional, feel happy and in love. Do not be afraid of your own emotions. Smile often and share joy and happiness.

Breathe and be grateful for being alive.

To make this exercise clearer, we will take an example. Think of Bereavement.

Bereavement

I to Identify

How many emotions can you identify?

Anger, sadness, sense of loss, fear, love, pain, resentfulness, guilt, regrets... Think, how many more?

Bereavement is not only one thing! It is complex, like the story of the elephant and how to break it into little pieces.

Why anger, perhaps you are angry with the deceased

because you feel abandoned, because he/she left before you. You may feel resentful because you are now with all the responsibilities of the household, etcetera, etcetera.

Sadness and sense of loss, because you will miss the person, there is a void, you are sad because you are not going to see the person again.

Fear because you will not know what is next, how are you going to cope.

Love because you feel you are still loving and caring for that person.

Pain as the loss is breaking your heart and you feel dying again and again every time your memory brings your loved one's death.

Guilt is perhaps one of the worst. As this feeling paralyses you. It keeps the pain inside like a knife digging in and in. When you feel responsible for what you did or something you did not do, when you feel you are the cause of harm, or you regret saying or doing something that it could be differently.

Guilt is the feeling of speculation, the king of IF! What if I said good bye and I was not angry at him when he died. What if I have done differently and perhaps if I had listened he would be alive... and so, and so.

Guilt will drive you nowhere as IF does not exist!

IF creates scenarios, mental exercises, hypothesis that are not healthy when we look into the past. What if I had done... It is a complete waste of time. You DID not Do it after the fact. When you were in the situation in that present moment you acted and that has a consequence. End of the story!

We need to learn to detach; therefore, to act in completely honesty and integrity, and if the outcome created a mistake or provide an opportunity to heal but in a painful way you can sincerely apologise and learn from your mistake. But, in that exact scenario, not IF I did this or that! Right there in the present, in the now of that specific situation.

Act in your present time, be mindful of your present, have a positive and selfless intention. When every step in our thinking is pure and transparent; when we act with integrity, the outcome can be faced and assumed in the same manner, even if it is painful or challenging.

You have to assume the responsibility of your acts, stop looking into the past and make amends when possible. No regrets, no guilt as they are mostly excuses. The only remedy to guilt is forgiveness, forgiveness of your own self.

O to Observe

Observe each one of that emotions inside of your body. Have a dialogue with them. Scan your body and find out where are they. Feel them with an open mind. Do not try to interpret them or to deny what you are seeing or feeling. Acknowledge them and listen to them. Honour them with no judgment.

T to Transform

Become one with your emotions, one by one you embrace them. You create a symbiotic relationship. You understand them and feel them intensely to become one. Associate them with something positive. Think in the qualities of the 9. Imagine you have the power to allocate them a new direction, to programme them with a positive input. Work with them as a team.

A to Accomplish

When that fusion is in there, feel it with love and compassion. Remember their new qualities, feel them, embrace them. Fused with love and gratitude. Then let them free. See them going around circulating vibrating full of life.

Be generous to your own self. Be grateful to your emotions, to your body who has stored them in a safe place until you were ready to deal with them. Feel that you have done it with integrity, love and deep compassion. Feel that the process is yours. It is no-body else's business. You can feel the sense of achievement.

S to Setting Free / Self-Realisation

Let me tell you a little Buddhist story:

There were two monks walking towards their monastery. They had been walking for days. One of them was an elderly man, a master, and the other was a cheerful, talkative young man who was under the tutelage of the elderly one. The young one was an obedient monk, enthusiastic and eager to learn.

On their path was a river they needed to cross. When they reached its banks, there was an attractive young woman in distress who was afraid of the water and could not swim. She urgently needed to cross the river and could not wait for anyone else to help her to go across.

Seeing her predicament, the elderly monk offered to carry her on his back across the river and the three of them crossed to the other side.

The girl was grateful to the monks for their help; she thanked them and said her goodbyes.

The monks carried on their walk and the young monk became quiet, serious, and pensive. He spent hours and hours pondering in his mind. They both walked until night and when they were near to their destination, suddenly the young man, not able to hold any longer, turned to his master and asked:

"Sir, why did you do that?" The elderly looked at him and said: " Did I do what?". "You know...that... You know it is against the rules to be in physical contact with a woman, and despite that you carried her." "Carried who?" The elderly replied.

"You know. The young, pretty lady at the river".

And the elderly replied: " I dropped her at the bank of the river; so, why are you still carrying her?"

When you embrace your emotions, when judgment ceases, when you are grateful and you have the sense of accomplishment. When you could not go any deeper to extract the last juices you can set it free. You can breathe out the energy that was stagnant. The energy that was crying for freedom.

When you feel that the emanation of these energies is coming out of yourself you feel that a transformation has been accomplished and now you are a new "ME".

People asked me: "How do you know? How do you know you are at that stage?" To what I reply: "You will feel it. You will not know. The clue is you will not have the need to ask for it"

My sweet darling, my beloved reader please do love your own self. You are kings and queens among royals. Your beauty is exceptional. The love you feel is sacred.

Please open up and feel your life flourishing spreading that love to all.

Nature is part of you, the seas, the sky, the mountains, the grass, the ladybirds. The trees, the sun, the pond, the ducks. The child's laugh, the sunrise, the darkness, the moon, the stars, the clouds. Love is contagious, love is life, love is beautiful, feel it and recognise it everywhere.

When you spread love, love comes back to you. You cannot love anyone or anything if you do not love yourself. As love is not being selfish, or being narcissistic, or egocentric. Love cannot be any of that, love is just love.

And last, please my beloved ones, think about your semantics. Words are not idle; they have a mental charge, an embedded emotion. They are codes, modems, CPUs with a purpose. Look at your language. Probably talk less in your inner dialogues and measure your language while talking to others. In doubt, check your dictionary, your thesaurus, analyse the word and what is its power of creation. Be a clear communicator; if your mind is organised, without bias, or providing misinterpretation; if there is integrity and honesty in your concepts, everything coming out from your mouth is a divine treasure.

Oh, WOW! Look at the time, we have been talking for hours. Time to go my sweet dear. Enough for now.

Have a lovely life; and remember:

The Healing process starts with YOU and ends with YOU.

Own your own healing!

Hasta la vista!

Adriana.

ABOUT THE AUTHOR

Adriana Kahrs was born in Bogota, Colombia and since she was a child, she was prone to put her hands on people, animals, and plants to make them better. Ever since, she had a heart full of compassion and intuition to be guided towards the areas where pain or other problems were.

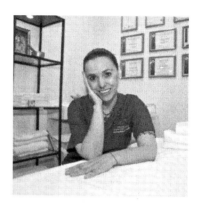

People were saying that they felt better; animals were healing. She was by then very intuitive and psychic, mainly about health issues. Time passed and she grew up and got experience in other sectors; she pursued a scientific career in Medicine, followed by Microbiology. After a few years she changed for an artistic approach with a career in Design, and later, explored a more commercial and managerial sector in Export Management.

In 2006, she studied Alternative and Complementary Therapies and enhanced her natural gifted abilities. Subsequently, she had the opportunity to create her dream; a clinic of different disciplines of alternative and complementary therapies, where they combine energy healing with therapeutic manual treatments and mind therapies, such as psychotherapy and hypnotherapy, to name a few.

She created a space where people can heal, relax and learn to be better, happier and healthier. She has different specialties, but she is particularly fond of treating people who have cancer as she has witnessed how much she can help them. For her, helping others in palliative care is a very humbling experience, where there is so much love, and so much humanity.

Adriana is an intelligent, gifted, knowledgeable, experienced, spiritual and generous woman who cares dearly for others. Her vocation and devotion is to help you to heal and release pain, stress and suffering. She is committed and dedicates her life to serve others with love, compassion and honesty.

To know more about me or my team please, visit our website: **www.spatiumclinic.co.uk**

Printed in Great Britain
by Amazon